100 Questions & Answers About Hydrocephalus

Aaron Mohanty, MD

Assistant Professor of Neurosurgery
University of Texas Medical Branch at Galveston
Galveston, Texas
Pediatric Neurosurgeon
Clearlake Regional Medical Center
Webster, Texas

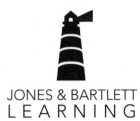

JONES & BARTLETT
L E A R N I N G

World Headquarters

Jones & Bartlett Learning
5 Wall Street
Burlington, MA 01803
978-443-5000
info@jblearning.com
www.jblearning.com

Jones & Bartlett Learning
Canada
6339 Ormindale Way
Mississauga, Ontario L5V 1J2
Canada

Jones & Bartlett Learning
International
Barb House, Barb Mews
London W6 7PA
United Kingdom

Jones & Bartlett Learning books and products are available through most bookstores and online booksellers. To contact Jones & Bartlett Learning directly, call 800-832-0034, fax 978-443-8000, or visit our website, www.jblearning.com.

Substantial discounts on bulk quantities of Jones & Bartlett Learning publications are available to corporations, professional associations, and other qualified organizations. For details and specific discount information, contact the special sales department at Jones & Bartlett Learning via the above contact information or send an email to specialsales@jblearning.com.

The authors, editor, and publisher have made every effort to provide accurate information. However, they are not responsible for errors, omissions, or for any outcomes related to the use of the contents of this book and take no responsibility for the use of the products and procedures described. Treatments and side effects described in this book may not be applicable to all people; likewise, some people may require a dose or experience a side effect that is not described herein. Drugs and medical devices are discussed that may have limited availability controlled by the Food and Drug Administration (FDA) for use only in a research study or clinical trial. Research, clinical practice, and government regulations often change the accepted standard in this field. When consideration is being given to use of any drug in the clinical setting, the health care provider or reader is responsible for determining FDA status of the drug, reading the package insert, and reviewing prescribing information for the most up-to-date recommendations on dose, precautions, and contraindications, and determining the appropriate usage for the product. This is especially important in the case of drugs that are new or seldom used.

Production Credits

Executive Publisher: Christopher Davis
Special Projects Editor: Kathy Richardson
Associate Editor: Laura Burns
Production Editor: Leah Corrigan
Associate Marketing Manager: Katie Hennessy
Manufacturing and Inventory Control
   Supervisor: Amy Bacus

Composition: Lynn L'Heureux
Cover Design: Carolyn Downer
Cover Image: © Monkey Business Images/
   ShutterStock, Inc.
Printing and Binding: Malloy, Inc.
Cover Printing: Malloy, Inc.

Library of Congress Cataloging-in-Publication Data
Mohanty, Aaron.
  100 questions & answers about hydrocephalus / Aaron Mohanty. -- 1st ed.
    p. cm.
  Includes bibliographical references and index.
  ISBN 978-0-7637-7990-0 (alk. paper)
  1. Hydrocephalus--Miscellanea. I. Title. II. Title: 100 questions and answers about hydrocephalus. III. Title: One hundred questions & answers about hydrocephalus.
  RC391.M64 2012
  616.85'8843--dc23

                    2011023284

6048

Printed in the United States of America
15 14 13 12 11 10 9 8 7 6 5 4 3 2 1

DEDICATION

This book is dedicated to my parents and my family for their encouragement, guidance, and tolerance.

A special dedication to all the children with hydrocephalus who have encouraged me to strive toward a better outcome.

—AM

CONTENTS

Contents

Hydrocephalus is one of the commonly encountered conditions in neuro-surgical practice. It is manifested by an excessive amount of cerebrospinal fluid in the brain compartments. Although it can affect any age group, it is commonly encountered either early or late in life. It has been estimated that the prevalence of congenital and infantile hydrocephalus ranges between 0.48 to 0.81 per 1,000 live and stillbirths. Hydrocephalus is frequently associated with other congenital anomalies, including spina bifida. Similarly, it has been well recognized that a subtype of hydrocephalus known as normal pressure hydrocephalus is widely prevalent among the geriatric population. A recent study estimated that as high as 9% to 14% of patients in assisted living and extended care suffer from idiopathic normal pressure hydrocephalus.

Hydrocephalus has been conventionally managed by inserting a ventricu-loperitoneal shunt. The shunt drains the fluid from the ventricular cavity to the abdominal cavity. Although shunts have been lifesaving in hydrocepha-lus, patients ultimately become shunt dependent. As mechanical devices, shunts can malfunction, and under such circumstances, emergency revision is warranted.

Thus, patients with hydrocephalus require constant follow-up and medi-cal attention. Families and caregivers need to be well acquainted with the diagnosis, treatment options, associated long-term dysfunctions, and overall outcome. More important, they need to identify the symptoms early to seek medical attention. This is significant because many patients demonstrate subtle delayed cognitive deficits and may not be able to indicate the symp-toms to require early attention.

This book essentially describes various types of hydrocephalus, their symp-toms, associated radiologic findings, and available management options for patients with this chronic condition. Considerable attention is devoted to available surgical management options. Commonly asked questions are answered with straightforward scientific explanations. This book attempts to bridge the gap between highly trained neuroscientists and those who are not medically trained but have several questions.

This book is intended for families and caregivers of patients with hydrocephalus who want to familiarize themselves with the condition and its symptoms. In addition, it will serve as a useful resource for paramedical staff, such as nurses, physician assistants, clinical psychologists, social workers, physiotherapists, and medical students, who are often involved in the management of these patients.

In simple terms, the purpose of this book can be summarized as *it answers everything that you wanted to ask your doctor but forgot during the appointment.*

Aaron Mohanty, MD

Mary M. George, PhD, completed her PhD in neuropsychology at the National Institute of Mental Health and Neurosciences at Bangalore, India, and subsequently completed a postdoctoral degree at Rice University, Houston, Texas. She is currently an Assistant Professor of Pediatrics at Baylor College of Medicine and a Pediatric Neuropsychologist at Texas Children's Hospital in Houston, Texas.

PART ONE

Introduction

What are hydrocephalus and cerebrospinal fluid?

Why do people develop hydrocephalus? How common is hydrocephalus?

Can hydrocephalus be passed down from parent to child?

1. What are hydrocephalus and cerebrospinal fluid?

Accumulation of excessive amounts of cerebrospinal fluid in the intracranial compartment is known as **hydrocephalus**. As we will see later, this fluid can accumulate either outside the brain (on the brain surface) or inside brain compartments known as ventricles. Increased fluid in the intracranial compartment in the neonatal period causes enlargement of the head size, thus leading to a large head in infants and in young children.

Cerebrospinal fluid (CSF, also commonly known as "spinal fluid") is the fluid encasing the brain and filling the crevices on the brain surface. It also fills the spaces inside the brain compartment known as ventricles. CSF extends into the spinal canal to surround the spinal cord and the nerve roots. The CSF supports the brain (many consider the brain to literally "float" in CSF), acts as a cushion by protecting it against external trauma, removes the metabolic wastes that the brain produces, and distributes biologically active substances throughout the brain.

2. Why do people develop hydrocephalus? How common is hydrocephalus?

Although we do not know exactly why some people develop hydrocephalus, we know how it happens in some of the people who have it. In the following chapters, we will go into more details about hydrocephalus.

It is very difficult to establish the incidence of hydrocephalus. The incidence of congenital hydrocephalus (hydrocephalus present at birth or that develops from a process before birth) has been found in 0.66 per 1,000 live births (6.6 per 10,000 births) in a recent study from Sweden. Assuming an average incidence of 5 per 10,000 births, an estimated 2,000 babies are born with congenital hydrocephalus every year in the United States.

Hydrocephalus

A medical condition in which there is an abnormal accumulation of cerebrospinal fluid in the ventricles or cavities of the brain.

Cerebrospinal fluid (CSF)

The clear bodily fluid present in the subarachnoid space (the space between the arachnoid mater and the pia mater) and the ventricular system. It acts as a "cushion" for the brain and provides a basic mechanical and immunologic protection to the brain inside the skull. CSF is produced in the choroid plexus.

3. Can hydrocephalus be passed down from parent to child?

Most types of hydrocephalus occur sporadically and is not inherited. However, a certain type of aqueductal stenosis known as X-linked aqueductal stenosis has been found to be inherited. This occurs only in males and has been found to be transmitted from one to the next by a female carrier (from mother to son). This is an extremely rare condition and has been found to occur in less than 2% of congenital hydrocephalus. Often, in addition to hydrocephalus, children have other anomalies of the brain (hypoplasia of the corticospinal tract, agenesis of corpus callosum, fusion of thalami).

In a recent study, 8% of patients with hydrocephalus reported a family history of hydrocephalus, and 3% described a first-degree relative who also suffered from the condition (Gupta, 2007).

Introduction

PART TWO

Anatomy of the Brain

Can you explain the basic anatomy of the brain?

How is CSF produced, and how does it circulate?
What are ventricles?

What is a suture?

Meninges

Membranes that envelop the central nervous system. The meninges consist of three layers: the outer dura mater, the middle arachnoid mater, and the deep pia mater. The primary function of the meninges is to cover and protect the central nervous system.

Dura mater

The outermost of the three layers of the meninges surrounding the brain and spinal cord (the other two meningeal layers are the pia mater and the arachnoid mater). The dura surrounds the brain and extends to cover the spinal cord.

Arachnoid mater

The middle of the three membranes that cover the brain and spinal cord.

Pia mater

The innermost layer of the three layers of membranes surrounding the brain and spinal cord.

To understand the various causes of hydrocephalus and the treatment options, we need to know the relevant brain anatomy, the cerebrospinal fluid pathways, and its normal circulation. Also, while trying to know more about hydrocephalus, it is natural to come across terminology relating to the brain. Hence, it is essential that we discuss the related anatomy of the brain.

4. Can you explain the basic anatomy of the brain?

Beneath the skull bone, the brain is covered by several layers of membranes, which, as a group, are known as **meninges**. From outside to inside, the membranes are **dura mater**, **arachnoid mater,** and **pia mater**. The dura is the toughest of all and is densely adherent to the overlying bone. It is so tightly attached that, at the time of surgery, the neurosurgeon has to strip it off from the bone. Thus, under normal circumstances, there is no space between the bone and the dura, though, at times, blood and pus can dissect through and develop an epidural space.

Beneath the dura lies the arachnoid mater (or, simply, arachnoid), which is composed of thin strands of tissues often coursing across the layer. Between the dura and the arachnoid lies the subdural space, which is a true space. Accumulation of blood, pus, or even CSF in the subdural space can occur easily and is named as subdural hematoma (blood), subdural empyema (pus), or subdural hygroma (CSF). Underneath the arachnoid layer is the subarachnoid space, which contains the CSF. Accumulation of blood in the subdural space is known as subarachnoid hemorrhage, which is often encountered after ruptured aneurysms. Unlike the epidural and subdural spaces, bleeding in the subarachnoid space usually does not clot well, as CSF prevents its clotting. Infection in the subarachnoid space is commonly known as meningitis.

Underneath the arachnoid and very closely attached to the brain surface is the very thin pia mater (or pia). The pia sticks to the brain surface and is difficult to separate, even with the operating microscope.

Compartments of the Cranial Cavity

The cranial cavity (also known in common terms as the skull) is divided into two major compartments by a thick structure known as the **tentorium cerebelli** (tentorium means shaped like a tent; cerebelli relates to cerebellum, the structure toward the back of the head that controls coordination; see later). It is composed of a double layer of dura mater, which is folded on itself and basically supports the brain superior to it (**Figure 1**). It also forms a support for the blood vessels and the nerves that course within it. The cranial compartments are known as **supratentorial** (on top of the tent) and **infratentorial compartment** (below the tent). The supra- and infratentorial compartments communicate by the tentorial notch, which accommodates the midbrain.

Tentorium cerebelli

An extension of the dura mater separating the cerebellum from the occipital lobes. It divides the cranial cavity into two major compartments: the supratentorial (above the tentorium) and infratentorial (below the tentorium) compartment.

Supratentorial compartment

The area located above the tentorium cerebelli. The supratentorial region contains the cerebral hemisphere.

Infratentorial compartment

The area located below the tentorium cerebelli. The infratentorial region contains the cerebellum and the brain stem.

Anatomy of the Brain

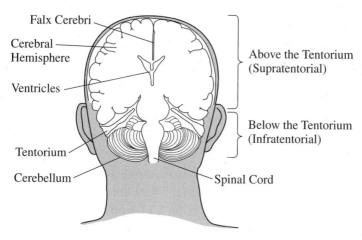

Falx Cerebri
Cerebral Hemisphere
Ventricles
Tentorium
Cerebellum
Above the Tentorium (Supratentorial)
Below the Tentorium (Infratentorial)
Spinal Cord

Figure 1. Compartments of the Cranial Cavity.

Adapted from "The brain." CancerHelp UK. http://www.cancerhelp.org.uk/type/brain-tumour/about/the-brain. Accessed February 24, 2011.

Cerebral hemisphere

One of two halves of the supratentorial part of the brain delineated by a median fissure and the falx cerebri.

Falx cerebri

A strong, arched fold of dura mater descending vertically between the cerebral hemispheres.

Brain herniation

Occurs as the brain shifts across structures within the skull usually as a result of very high intracranial pressure. If not treated quickly, brain herniation can be fatal.

Frontal lobes

An area in the brain located in the front part of each cerebral hemisphere. They are positioned in front of the parietal lobes and above and in front of the temporal lobes.

Motor strip

A band of cerebral cortex (gray matter) running along the side of the frontal lobe of the brain that controls all bodily motor movements.

The major structures occupying the supratentorial compartment are the **cerebral hemispheres** (left and right) and the deeper nuclear structures (thalamus, basal ganglia). The major structures occupying the infratentorial compartment are the cerebellum (left and right) and the brain stem. Both cerebral hemispheres are divided again by a fold of dura mater known as **falx cerebri**. A very ill-formed falx cerebelli divides the right and left cerebellum.

As the cranial cavity is divided into several compartments that communicate with one another by relatively narrow passages, localized increased pressure in one compartment will tend to push the brain tissue to adjacent compartments with lower pressure. This is known as **brain herniation** and sometimes is seen in hydrocephalus. The displaced brain presses on normal brain tissues, impairing their function, and can often compress blood vessels supplying other areas of brain, leading to stroke and neurologic deficits.

Structure of the Brain

The supratentorial compartment of the brain houses the cerebral hemispheres and the deep brain structures. There are two cerebral hemispheres: left and right. Each hemisphere has four lobes (**Figure 2**). The **frontal lobes** are located in the front of the brain and above the eyeballs. The frontal lobes are very well developed in humans and account for thinking, judgment, reasoning, and other higher mental functions that differentiate humans from other animals. The motor area of the brain, which controls the movement of the opposite side of the body (i.e., the right frontal lobe controls the left hand and leg movements), is located toward the back part of the frontal lobes (approximately around the line joining both ears). This is known as the **motor strip**. In the motor strip, localization is arranged in a specific pattern: The face area is located down (behind and above the lateral angle of the eye), and the leg area is located higher (toward the top of the skull). A region of the frontal lobes known as **Broca's area** is responsible for

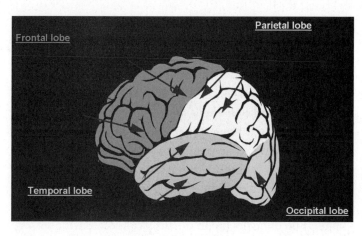

Figure 2. Lobes of the Brain.

Adapted from Netter FH. *The CIBA Collection of Medical Illustrations, Volume I: Nervous System.* CIBA Pharmaceutical Company, 1983, page 23, Section II, Plate 1.

Anatomy of the Brain

speech. Thinking logically, one can assume that Broca's area would be located in the region of facial representation in the motor strip, that is, behind and slightly superior to the outer angle of the eye. Behind the frontal lobes are the **parietal lobes,** which are responsible for appreciating sensation. The lower part of the parietal lobes is also responsible for speech coordination. Lying at the top of the ear are the **temporal lobes,** which have centers for comprehension and hearing. Toward the back of the head are the **occipital lobes,** which are responsible for vision.

As each side of the brain controls the opposite side of the body (motor, sensory, some of the vision and hearing), it is logical to assume that there are connections between both halves of brain. In fact, there are several connections, the most important of which is the **corpus callosum** (Figure 4 and Figure 15, p. 52). Corpus callosum is a thick band of fibers communicating between the right and left cerebral hemispheres (something like a freeway communicating between two large cities). The corpus callosum lies just above the lateral ventricles (see later), which contain CSF. In chronic hydrocephalus, the

Broca's area

A region of the brain in the lower and posterior part of the frontal lobe and is responsible for speech production. It is named after Paul Broca who first associated the area to speech production.

Parietal lobes

A part of the brain located above the temporal and occipital lobes and behind the frontal lobes.

Temporal lobes

The region of the brain cortex located in the temporal region behind the frontal lobes, beneath the parietal lobes and in front of the occiptial lobes.

Occipital lobes

Located in the back part of the brain behind the parietal lobes and contains the visual cortex and processing center.

Corpus callosum

A bundle of nerve fibers connecting the left and right cerebral hemispheres, thus transferring information between the two halves of the brain.

Internal capsule

A region of brain composed of white matter that separates the caudate nucleus and the thalamus from the lenticular nucleus.

Thalamus

A midline-paired structure situated between the cerebral cortex and brain stem.

Hypothalamus

The part of the brain below the thalamus that contains a number of small nuclei with a variety of functions.

Basal ganglia

A group of nuclei situated deep in the brain that are connected with the cerebral cortex, thalamus, and other areas.

Cerebellum

Located in the back part of the brain below the cerebral hemispheres.

Brain stem

The posterior part of the brain that is continuous with the spinal cord.

corpus callosum gets stretched and thinned out. In some types of congenital conditions (including congenital hydrocephalus), the corpus callosum is underdeveloped or even absent.

There are several densely packed structures toward the center of the brain. Some of these are compact fibers conducting impulses from the brain to the spinal cord, and others are a conglomeration of deep nuclei (nuclei are compact dense cells located in the brain). Some common ones are **internal capsule** (band of fibers transferring impulse to and from the brain to the spine and other regions), **thalamus** (dense conglomeration of nuclei predominantly connected with sensory and motor relays), **hypothalamus** (concerned with autonomic functions and endocrine functions), and **basal ganglia** (composed of several nuclei and concerned with movements and posture).

Infratentorial Compartment

The infratentorial compartment houses the cerebellum and brain stem. There are also several important cranial nerves that arise from the brain stem and pass through the posterior fossa as they exit from the cranial cavity. The **cerebellum** is composed of two cerebellar hemispheres and a midline vermis. Collectively, these are responsible for coordinating various synchronized body movements, including gait. As speech is also a coordinated movement between various muscle groups, speech disturbances also occur with cerebellar dysfunction. The **brain stem** is the most vital structure of the body and is responsible for respiration, cardiac function, and arousal. It also houses centers (nuclei) of various cranial nerves that control swallowing, bowel movements, respiration, and facial functions and sensation. The brain stem is divided into three regions: midbrain, pons, and medulla (from top to bottom).

The supratentorial compartment has three cavities, or ventricles: the two lateral ventricles (right and left) and the third ventricle, which is located in the midline (see next question). The fourth ventricle is located in the posterior fossa and is situated between the brain stem (in front) and the cerebellum (behind).

5. How is CSF produced, and how does it circulate? What are ventricles?

Most of the CSF is produced by a structure called **choroid plexus**. These are strands of tissue with a rich supply of blood vessels that actively secrete CSF. Normally, the CSF is produced at a rate of 0.35 milliliters per minute. For all practical purposes, about 500 milliliters (16 ounces) of CSF is produced every day. Considering that the average CSF volume is 150 milliliters, it is obvious that the CSF turns itself over three times every day.

The choroid plexus is located inside the brain cavities known as ventricles (**Figure 3** and **Figure 4**). There are four ventricles in the brain (two lateral ventricles, the right and left, one third ventricle, and one fourth ventricle). The bulk of the choroid plexus is located in both lateral ventricles. However, a small amount of choroid plexus is present in the third and fourth ventricles also. A small fraction of CSF is also produced by the ependymal lining (the thin layer of cells that lines the ventricles). As we will discuss later, this is why removal or cauterization of the choroid plexus does not result in complete control of hydrocephalus.

Once produced, CSF circulates through the ventricular system, which consists of the ventricles with narrow passages connecting to one another (Figures 3 and 4). From the most capacious lateral ventricles, CSF moves to the third ventricle through the **foramen of Monro** (sometimes spelled "Munro"). As there are two lateral ventricles, there are two foramina of Monro, one from each **lateral ventricle** connecting the third ventricle. The **third ventricle** is normally slitlike and is located

---

Anatomy of the Brain

Choroid plexus

A specialized cerebrospinal fluid–producing structure, is present in the lateral, third, and fourth ventricles.

Foramen of Monro

A channel that connects the lateral ventricle with the third ventricle and is located just next to the midline of the brain.

Lateral ventricles

Part of the ventricular system of the brain. There are two lateral ventricles, one on each side of the brain. They are the largest of the ventricles.

Third ventricle

Part of the ventricular system located between the two thalami in the midline.

For all practical purposes, about 500 milliliters (16 ounces) of CSF is produced every day.

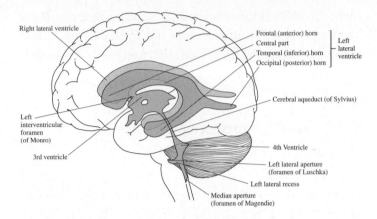

Figure 3. Diagrammatic Representation of the Ventricles of the Brain.

Adapted from Netter FH. *The CIBA Collection of Medical Illustrations, Volume I: Nervous System.* CIBA Pharmaceutical Company, 1983, page 30, Section II, Plate 8.

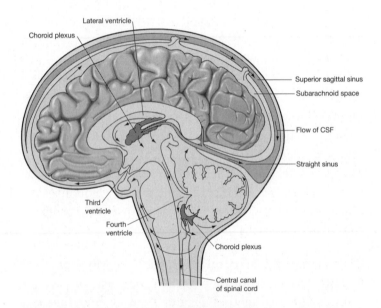

Figure 4. Sagittal Section of the Brain with the CSF Circulation.

Adapted from Netter FH. *The CIBA Collection of Medical Illustrations, Volume I: Nervous System.* CIBA Pharmaceutical Company, 1983, page 31, Section II, Plate 9.

exactly in the midline. It is surrounded on both sides by two well-formed structures—the thalamus and the hypothalamus, which is why the third ventricle does not dilate as much as the lateral ventricles when hydrocephalus develops. The floor of the third ventricle is formed by relatively thinner brain tissue, which contains some of the hypothalamic nuclei. Beneath the floor are located some of the important fluid-filled crevices (**cisterns**): the suprasellar cistern and the interpeduncular cistern, which contain many important blood vessels. As we will see later, many neurosurgeons use the relative thinness of the third ventricular floor to make a fenestration in diverting the CSF out of the ventricles in obstructive hydrocephalus.

The third ventricle communicates with the fourth ventricle by a very narrow passage: the **cerebral aqueduct** (also known as aqueduct of sylvius). The aqueduct is approximately 1 centimeter (less than 1/2 inch) long and is slightly angled toward the back of the head. As the narrowest part of the ventricular system, the aqueduct is the most common site for obstruction in the pathway.

The aqueduct leads into the **fourth ventricle,** which is surrounded by the brain stem in front and the cerebellum in the sides and back. The fourth ventricle contains a narrow strip of choroid plexus ion in the roof. The fourth ventricle opens into the subarachnoid spaces though one midline and two lateral foramina known as the **foramen of Magendie** and **foramen of Luschka**, respectively.

The subarachnoid spaces are the CSF-filled spaces that contain the cranial nerves exiting from the brain and the blood vessels supplying the brain. At places, the subarachnoid space dips into the crevices at the surface of the brain. These crevices are known as the subarachnoid cisterns and can be identified in conventional CT and MRI scans.

Anatomy of the Brain

Cisterns

Crevices in the subarachnoid space of the brain created by a separation of the arachnoid and pia mater filled with cerebrospinal fluid. There are many cisterns in the brain.

Cerebral aqueduct

A narrow channel that drains cerebrospinal fluid is located within the midbrain connecting the third ventricle to the fourth ventricle.

Fourth ventricle

One of the four fluid-filled cavities in the brain. It is located behind the brain stem in the region of the pons and medulla.

Foramen of Magendie

The median aperture communicating the fourth ventricle to the cisterna magna.

Foramen of Luschka

The lateral apertures, one on each side, communicating the fourth ventricle to the cisterna magna.

Cisterna magna (large cistern)

One of the largest cisterns surrounding the brain.

Arachnoid granulations

Also known as arachnoid villi; these are small protrusions of the arachnoid (the thin second layer covering the brain) through the dura mater (the outer layer).

Anterior fontanel

The largest fontanel, which is located just behind the forehead in the midline and is placed at the junction of the sagittal suture, coronal suture, and the metopic suture.

Craniosynostosis

A condition in which there is premature fusion of one or more sutures in an infant skull, thus changing the growth pattern of the skull.

The fourth ventricle opens into a large subarachnoid space known as the **cisterna magna** (large cistern). CSF from the cistern magna then flows into the spinal canal and over the surface of the brain. CSF circulates around the brain surface and finally gets absorbed into the bloodstream through the **arachnoid granulations** high on the surface of the brain (Figure 4). The granulations' pores, as we will see later, may get blocked by red blood cell products (in case of bleeding into the subarachnoid space) or by a high concentration of protein in the CSF. Some CSF also gets absorbed across the ependymal lining of the ventricles and from the spinal subarachnoid space.

6. What is a suture?

Cranial sutures are the small deficiencies between plates of skull bones in which one plate of skull bone joins with another (**Figure 5**). In the skull, as in rest of the body, bone formation occurs at several places simultaneously (known as ossification centers), which subsequently join together. As the bone grows, the island of areas deficient in bone slowly disappears. One island is quite large at birth and is known as the **anterior fontanel** (soft spot) (Figure 5). In hydrocephalus due to increased intracranial pressure, the sutures usually separate and are prominent. The sutural separation leads to an increase in head circumference. In a condition known as **craniosynostosis,** the sutures get abnormally fused, resulting in a smaller or a distorted head. To make things more complex, sometimes craniosynostosis can be associated with hydrocephalus, and in this situation, the head size usually is not enlarged.

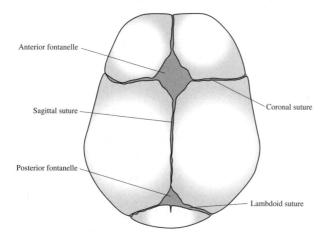

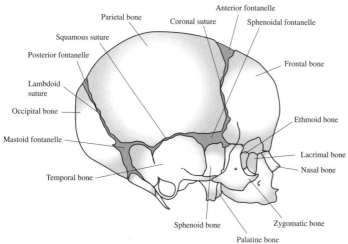

Figure 5.   Sutures of the Skull.

Adapted from Netter FH. *The CIBA Collection of Medical Illustrations, Volume I: Nervous System.* CIBA Pharmaceutical Company, 1983, page 10, Section I, Plate 8.

Anatomy of the Brain

PART THREE

Types of Hydrocephalus

How do you differentiate between obstructive hydrocephalus and communicating hydrocephalus?

How does congenital hydrocephalus differ from acquired hydrocephalus?

What is arrested hydrocephalus, and how does it differ from compensated hydrocephalus?

More...

Although, in broad terms, hydrocephalus means excessive accumulation of CSF in the brain, depending on the site of accumulation, the nature of hydrocephalus differs. The presentation and treatment options of the various types of hydrocephalus vary, depending on the location, rapidity of development of the accumulation, and the age of the patient.

7. How do you differentiate between obstructive hydrocephalus and communicating hydrocephalus?

Often one comes across a report by a radiologist or a neurosurgeon that adds the term *communicating* or *obstructive* before *hydrocephalus*. These terms were coined several decades ago to explain whether obstructed ventricular CSF communicated with subarachnoid CSF. To elaborate, if the obstruction is at or proximal to the fourth ventricular outlet foramina (foramen of Magendie and Luschka), then it is an **obstructive hydrocephalus** (**Figure 6**). However, if the obstruction is beyond the fourth ventricular outlet foramina (say, at the cisterns or arachnoid granulations), it is called **communicating hydrocephalus**. When the term was initially coined, it considered the results based on the investigations available then (ventriculogram, pneumoencephalogram). With the arrival of CT and MRI, those investigations were no longer necessary in most cases. The terms *communicating* and *obstructive* became outdated though not obsolete. However, as we will see later, a recent therapeutic procedure called the endoscopic third ventriculostomy has generated renewed interest in these terms.

8. How does congenital hydrocephalus differ from acquired hydrocephalus?

Hydrocephalus present at birth is known as **congenital hydrocephalus**. At times, congenital hydrocephalus is apparent a few weeks or months after birth, although the processes that

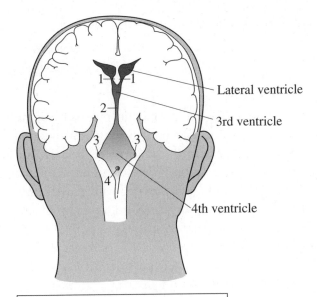

1. Interventircular foramina (of Monro)
2. Cere aqueduct (of Sylvius)
3. Lateral apertures (of Luschka)
4. Median aperture (of Magendie)

Figure 6. Possible Sites of CSF Obstruction in Hydrocephalus.

Adapted from Netter FH. *The CIBA Collection of Medical Illustrations, Volume I: Nervous System.* CIBA Pharmaceutical Company, 1983, page 8, Section I, Plate 6.

caused it evolved when the child was in the uterus. Congenital hydrocephalus is commonly obstructive. Intrauterine infections, such as toxoplasmosis (a parasite) or cytomegalovirus (CMV; a virus), can also cause congenital hydrocephalus.

Acquired hydrocephalus, as the name suggests, indicates the cause occurred sometime after the child was born. Some causes of acquired hydrocephalus include posttraumatic hydrocephalus, hydrocephalus associated with tumors, and normal pressure hydrocephalus.

Acquired hydrocephalus

Hydrocephalus caused by conditions that are not present at birth.

9. My doctor mentioned to me that my husband has chronic hydrocephalus. What does it signify? How does it differ from acute hydrocephalus?

These terminologies usually imply the rapid development of hydrocephalus. Hydrocephalus that develops within days or a few weeks is usually termed acute hydrocephalus. It is manifested by a rapid progression of symptoms and requires urgent treatment. Hydrocephalus associated with tumors obstructing the CSF pathway is an example of acute hydrocephalus. However, a slow progression of symptoms over months or even years is termed *chronic hydrocephalus*. As we will see later, chronic hydrocephalus usually presents with subtle signs of memory impairment, walking difficulty, or urinary incontinence. A classic example of chronic hydrocephalus is **normal pressure hydrocephalus,** which is usually seen in the geriatric population. At times, chronic hydrocephalus can present acutely due to a change in the pathophysiology of CSF absorption or flow.

10. What is arrested hydrocephalus and how does it differ from compensated hydrocephalus?

Arrested hydrocephalus: This represents a condition in which the ventricles are large, and the patient has no significant symptoms to require a surgical procedure. However, use this term with caution, as it is well known that these patients may develop symptoms very slowly and over a prolonged period. Sometimes they may manifest acutely, following a precipitating event such as minor trauma or infection, which alters the CSF dynamics.

Compensated hydrocephalus: Compensated hydrocephalus refers to a patient with enlarged ventricles, with a nonfunctional shunt or in whom the shunt has been removed. Although the majority of these patients do not demonstrate

Normal pressure hydrocephalus (NPH)

Commonly seen in elderly people, this form of communicating hydrocephalus presents with a varying combination of memory impairment, gait instability, and urinary incontinence.

gross symptoms, most will improve to a certain extent with shunt.

Often, it is difficult to differentiate between the two terminologies, leading some neurologists or neurosurgeons to use these terms interchangeably, adding to the confusion.

Types of Hydrocephalus

PART FOUR

Recognizing Hydrocephalus

How do infants and younger children with hydrocephalus present?

What is the anterior fontanel (soft spot)?
What should I look for in the soft spot?

Can a person with hydrocephalus have seizures?

More...

In hydrocephalus, CSF is retained inside the cranial compartment, resulting in increased intracranial pressure and dilatation of ventricles. This causes compression of the adjacent brain, resulting in clinical symptoms. The symptoms differ considerably in different age groups. In infants, a thin and relatively nonrigid skull allows for an expansion, while in adults and older children, the rigid and fused skull prevents expansion. We will briefly discuss the symptoms encountered in each category.

In hydrocephalus, CSF is retained inside the cranial compartment, resulting in increased intracranial pressure and dilatation of ventricles.

11. How do infants and younger children with hydrocephalus present?

In congenital hydrocephalus, either the infant is born with a large head or the head circumference abnormally grows during the first few months of life. If the child has an associated spinal defect, it is evident. The anterior fontanel (soft spot) is usually full; it may or may not bulge. In extreme cases, a relatively higher intracranial pressure allows blood to divert from the intracranial to the extracranial compartment, resulting in prominent and dilated scalp veins. A late feature is the classic "sunset sign" manifested by downward deviation of the eyeballs (resembling a setting sun). This is due to compression of the center of the upward eye movements located in the upper part of the brain stem (known as tectum) by the posterior part of the dilated third ventricle. In later stages, the child will be unduly irritable, fussy, and unable to eat. It may be associated with vomiting. Usually, there is no associated fever or diarrhea. Lethargy, drowsiness, and, in extreme cases, coma will follow if the child remains untreated.

12. Why does my pediatrician measure the head size every time my baby goes to see her? What is the head circumference chart? Can you make me understand how the chart is plotted and how it should be interpreted?

Head circumference (occipitofrontal circumference [OFC]): The pediatrician records the baby's head size in addition to the height and weight. Although there are no set points as to where the head should be measured, the largest diameter involving the **nasion** (the area above the root of the nose in the forehead) and the **inion** (occipital prominence, the midline prominence in the back of the head) is measured. Sometimes, the measurement varies even when the same person takes the measurement on different occasions. Hence, in cases of inconsistencies, the largest diameter is usually recorded. The measurement is plotted on the head circumference chart. Normally, the head grows along a curve: the 50th percentile—the solid line in the graph (**Figure 7** and **Figure 8**). However, as elsewhere in medicine, there is usually a range for normal head circumference (the dashed 5th and 95th percentile lines) (Figures 7 and 8). When your doctor plots the head circumference, he looks at the following parameters:

Nasion

The nasion lies in the intersection of the frontal the nasal bones. It is identified by the depressed area between the eyes, just superior to the root of the nose.

Inion

The inion is the most prominent projection of the occipital bone at the lower back part of the skull.

1. If the initial head circumference is within the 5th and the 95th percentiles (between the dashed lines)

2. If the head circumference matches appropriately with the rest of the parameters (height and weight)

3. If the head circumference measurements stays within the range during subsequent visits

4. If the child's head circumference growth curve runs parallel with the lines in the growth chart

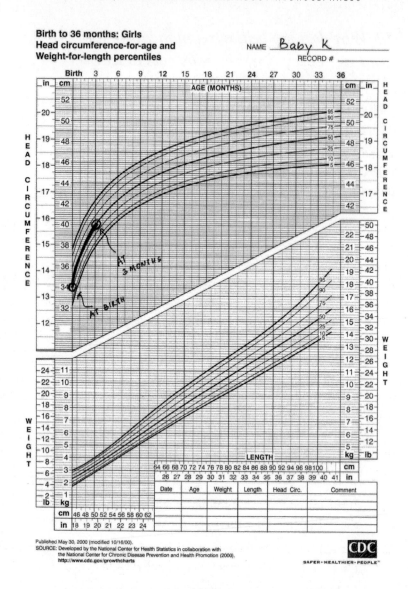

Birth to 36 months: Girls
Head circumference-for-age and
Weight-for-length percentiles

NAME _Baby K_

RECORD # _____

Published May 30, 2000 (modified 10/16/00).
SOURCE: Developed by the National Center for Health Statistics in collaboration with
the National Center for Chronic Disease Prevention and Health Promotion (2000).
http://www.cdc.gov/growthcharts

Figure 7. Growth Chart Showing Head Growth in a Normal Child.

Developed by the National Center for Health Statistics in collaboration with
the National Center for Chronic Disease Prevention and Health Promotion
(2000). http://www.cdc.gov/growthcharts, as modified.

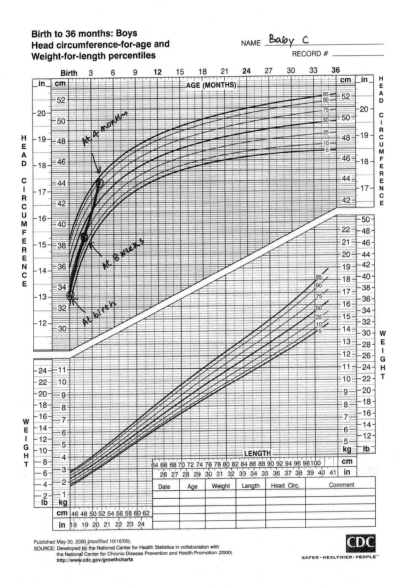

Birth to 36 months: Boys
Head circumference-for-age and
Weight-for-length percentiles

NAME Baby C

RECORD #

Figure 8. Growth Chart Demonstrating Abnormal Head Growth in a Child.

Developed by the National Center for Health Statistics in collaboration with the National Center for Chronic Disease Prevention and Health Promotion (2000). http://www.cdc.gov/growthcharts, as modified.

For example, Baby Girl K, a healthy female baby, was born uneventfully at 38 weeks of pregnancy with a head circumference of 34 centimeters at birth (Figure 7). At 3 months of age, the head circumference was 40 centimeters, and at 5 months of age, the head circumference was 43 centimeters. If we plot the growth, one would realize that the head is growing appropriate for the age as (a) the measurements have stayed within the curve, and (b) the line plotted by joining the measurement is parallel to the curve, that is, not pointing up or becoming flat.

Now, let us have an example of Baby Boy C who was born full term with a head circumference of 33 centimeters (Figure 8). At 8 weeks of age, the head circumference was 38.5 centimeters, and at 4 months of age, it measured 44 centimeters. If we plot the head growth in the chart (for boys), one would realize that the curve points more upward than the age-appropriate curve. This indicates that the child will require further investigations, such as a head ultrasound or CT scan for an inappropriately enlarging head.

The average head circumference in term infants measures around 35 centimeters. It increases approximately 1 centimeter every month during the first year of life, with the most rapid growth occurring during the first 6 months. The growth slows for the second year, with the head circumference on an average increasing by only 2 centimeters. Similarly, the brain is approximately two thirds of its ultimate adult size by the end of the first year of life, while by the end of second year, it grows up to four fifths of its ultimate adult size. Normally, the head circumference is plotted every 6–8 weeks unless indicated otherwise. The growth chart for boys differs from the growth chart for girls of similar age.

13. What is the anterior fontanel (soft spot)? What should I look for in the soft spot?

The soft spot on the top of head is the area where the bone is deficient in a newborn or in a child younger than 1 year

(Figure 5, p. 15). This is a normal phenomenon, and the deficient bone site is actually where the bone grows as the child ages. The soft spot is a useful "window" in this age group that reflects the intracranial pressure of the brain noninvasively. We lose this opportunity in older children and adults because the bone fills the space usually between 6 months and 18 months of age (see Question 6, p. 14).

Normally, when the child is quiet and positioned erect (e.g., while taking a nap in mom's arms with the head elevated), the soft spot is lax and below the margins of the adjacent bone. The bone margins can be easily felt. Under normal circumstances, crying will make the anterior fontanel full because crying, irritability, or coughing increases the intracranial pressure, reflected in fullness of the soft spot. However, in hydrocephalus, the increased intracranial pressure causes the soft spot to bulge even when the child is sleeping or quiet. Therefore, the status of the soft spot is ideally evaluated when the child is resting with the head elevated.

We lose this opportunity in older children and adults because the bone fills the space usually between 6 months and 18 months of age.

14. How do adults and older children with hydrocephalus present?

In this age group, fusion of the skull bones no longer permits the cranium to enlarge. The enlarging ventricles result in raised intracranial pressure and cause compression of the adjacent brain. There are two common modes of presentation:

1. Rapidly progressive hydrocephalus

2. Chronic hydrocephalus

In the first group, the increasing CSF accumulation increases the intracranial pressure, which presents with new onset headache and vomiting. These are commonly known as features of raised intracranial pressure. (You may hear these terms during discussion with your doctor.) If untreated, these symptoms worsen and blurry vision may occur. In chronic hydrocephalus, patients can develop diminution of vision as transmission of pressure from the intracranial compartment affects the optic nerve (nerve of vision). If still untreated, patients become drowsy and progress to coma, which happens relatively quicker in adults than in infants. Fused skull bones in adults cannot expand, thus preventing dampening effects that would otherwise have occurred by the expanding skull. Usually limb weakness is not experienced, although walking difficulty or the sensation of the knees giving way can occur. This happens because the motor fibers supplying leg muscles are placed next to the ventricles, and with the dilatation of the ventricles, fibers are stretched causing mild weakness.

At times, CSF accumulates slowly over months to years. This type of presentation is mostly seen in the elderly age group, although it can happen in younger ages. The patient becomes progressively dull, apathetic, and uninvolved with his or her surroundings. Memory impairment of recent events is common; usually, remote memory is well preserved. Walking difficulty, with short steps, a broad stance, and unsteadiness, is apparent. Urinary incontinence is also observed. Initially, the patient experiences urgency of micturition (having to rush to the bathroom), but in late stages, it progresses to incontinence and dribbling of urine. It is uncertain why these patients do not have significant headache as the ventricles dilate. It is assumed that slow dilatation of the ventricles compresses the adjacent brain to accommodate for extra fluid without causing raised pressure.

15. Can a person with hydrocephalus have seizures?

Seizures (also known as convulsions, or fits) occur because of excitatory phenomenon affecting some of the brain cells. The impulse travels rapidly, stimulating nearby cells and resulting in jerky movements or numbness of the opposite limbs. Seizures are caused by a focal, or localized, excitatory phenomenon in the brain. Because hydrocephalus is a more generalized condition, it uncommonly presents with seizures. However, seizures can

Seizures

Also known as a "fit," seizure is defined in medical literature as a transient symptom of abnormal excessive or synchronous neuronal activity in the brain.

result because of the pathology responsible for hydrocephalus (tumor, head injury) rather than because of the hydrocephalus.

In patients with obstructive hydrocephalus, one important symptom can mimic seizure activity, but if the patient is misdiagnosed, it can be devastating or even fatal. This happens during the later stage of hydrocephalus and has been known as *cerebellar fits*, or *hydrocephalic attacks*. In order not to confuse them with seizures, I prefer hydrocephalic attack. Usually, the patient lapses into sudden unconsciousness, which is typically preceded by progressively severe headaches. The lower limbs may stiffen, and the upper limbs may flex at the elbows or straighten. The eyeballs are usually directed downward. The condition can be associated with respiratory disturbances. The patient remains in this stage for a few seconds to minutes. Often, the patient recovers spontaneously in a few minutes, but the symptoms recur till the hydrocephalus is relieved. This condition is associated with significant morbidity and can be uniformly fatal unless prompt CSF drainage is instituted. This is a true medical emergency, and under no circumstances should the treatment be delayed.

The most common explanation is that rapid increase in intracranial pressure pushes the brain downward, causing the herniating brain to impinge on the brain stem. Centers for respiration, blood pressure, consciousness, and other vital functions are located in the brain stem, and impairment of the brain stem function can cause sudden respiratory arrest and death.

Some patients who develop herniation but were saved by immediate CSF drainage may develop blindness in half of the visual field (visual field defects). This happens as the blood vessels supplying the occipital lobes are trapped and compressed by the herniating brain, leading to infarction (stroke) of the occipital lobes. Once developed, it is usually permanent even with successful management of hydrocephalus.

PART FIVE

Hydrocephalus Associated with Specific Conditions

What is the relationship of hydrocephalus to spina bifida?

Can hydrocephalus occur after severe trauma to the brain?

What are the other conditions associated with hydrocephalus?

More...

16. What is the relationship of hydrocephalus to spina bifida?

Spina bifida essentially means a split, or a bifid, spine. It indicates a condition wherein the child is born with a defect in the low or midback associated with weakness and exposed neural tissue, commonly known as lumbar **myelomeningocele**. Several types of spina bifida vary in severity and involvement; however, we will focus on lumbar myelomeningocele, as this is the most common type of spina bifida. Most of these children will have associated hydrocephalus. Although only one fourth (25%) of children with myelomeningocele have associated hydrocephalus at birth, almost 80% of children with lumbar myelomeningocele will ultimately develop hydrocephalus and will require surgery. The incidence is less than for other types of spina bifida. A combination of several factors cause hydrocephalus in children with lumbar myelomeningocele; however, it is usually associated with a condition known as **Chiari malformation** (descent of part of the cerebellum, known as the tonsils, into the upper part of the spinal cord in the neck) and the associated deformity of the brain stem, which obstructs the CSF flow.

Conventionally, if a child is born with an open spinal defect and has associated hydrocephalus, the neurosurgeon will initially repair the open defect within 1 or 2 days of birth. There is some controversy about timing the placement of the shunt. Some will consider ventricular taps (see later) to temporarily drain the CSF from the ventricles every day or every alternate day for several days. Subsequently, a shunt insertion is considered. This schedule allows avoiding placing the shunt when the myelomeningocele is repaired. Studies have shown the risk of shunt infection is least if the shunt placement is delayed for a few days after the repair. In a previous report, 83% of shunts became infected when placed before the repair, 23% had a shunt infection when both surgeries were done simultaneously, and only 7.3% had a shunt infection when

Myelomeningocele

In this form of spina bifida, through a defect in the coverings of the spinal cord (either all or some of the following: meninges, muscle, bone, skin) the neural tissue (spinal cord or the nerve roots) protrude outside the confinement of the spinal canal in varying degrees.

Chiari malformation

In Chiari malformation, there is a downward displacement of the cerebellar tonsils into the upper part of the spinal canal through the foramen magnum.

the shunt was placed after the repair. However, others will consider placing the shunt at the same time as the repair, basing their decision on other studies that found significant differences in infection rates.

Karen's comment:

When Joshua was born, he had an open spina bifida that needed to be surgically closed on the same day. At birth, he had a normal head size, but the doctors told us that most likely he would develop hydrocephalus and would require a shunt. We took Josh for a checkup every 2 weeks, and the doctors would measure his head circumference and repeat CT scans every 2 to 3 months. Surprisingly, Josh did not develop hydrocephalus that would require surgery. He has a very mild form of hydrocephalus, which the doctors tell us is pretty stable. He is in fifth grade now and gets all A's on school tests.

17. What is Dandy–Walker malformation?

Dandy-Walker malformation is a clinical condition associated with congenital obstruction of the fourth ventricular outlet, hydrocephalus, and inadequate development (hypoplasia) of the cerebellar vermis (**Figure 9**). Considering that it is associated with obstruction at the fourth ventricular outlet foramina, Dandy-Walker malformation is a type of obstructive hydrocephalus manifesting with dilatation of the fourth ventricle, third ventricle, and often the lateral ventricles. It accounts for 2–4% of all hydrocephalus. Apart from manifesting with a large head, these children have been found to have multiple intracranial anomalies. Associated abnormalities of **corpus callosum** (commonly nonformation or partial formation) are apparent in 17% of children. Other additional anomalies include facial abnormalities (cleft palate, angioma), ocular abnormalities (micropthalmia, retinal dysgenesis), and cardiac abnormalities (patent ductus arteriosus, septal defects). There can also be a host of central nervous system abnormalities, including occipital encephalocele, syringomyelia, and spinal

Dandy-Walker malformation

A congenital brain malformation involving the cerebellum and the fourth ventricle. The components of Dandy-Walker syndrome include absence of cerebellar vermis, obstruction of the opening of the fourth ventricle, and associated hydrocephalus. All components may or may not be present. There may be various degrees of associated developmental delay. It is considered to be a genetically sporadic disorder that occurs in 1 in every 25,000 live births.

Corpus callosum

A bundle of nerve fibers connecting the left and right cerebral hemispheres, thus transferring information between the two halves of the brain.

abnormalities. Various degree of intellectual impairment is seen in approximately half of the patients. About 15% have associated seizures.

The accepted treatment for Dandy-Walker malformation is placing a shunt either from the lateral ventricle (**ventriculo-peritoneal shunt**) or from the fourth ventricle (**cystoperito-neal shunt**, although it is called cystoperitoneal, it drains from the dilated fourth ventricle). Some surgeons place a shunt from both the lateral and the fourth ventricle and connect the proximal ends by a **Y connector** to drain into a single distal tube. In recent years, endoscopic third ventriculostomy has also been effective.

Ventriculo-peritoneal shunt

A shunt that drains CSF between the cerebral ventricles and the peritoneal cavity (also known as abdominal cavity). The peritoneum is the lining of the abdominal cavity.

Cystoperitoneal shunt

A shunt placed between the cyst (fluid cavity) in the brain and the abdominal cavity.

Y connector

A connector commonly used with cerebral shunts to connect two ventricular ends (one each to the upper limbs of the Y) to a single distal end (the lower limb of the Y).

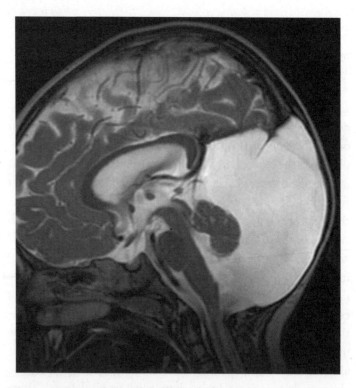

Figure 9. MRI in Dandy Walker Malformation. Note the large cyst in the brain in the back.

18. Can hydrocephalus occur after severe trauma to the brain?

Hydrocephalus can also develop following a severe head injury. It can occur in two settings, acute hydrocephalus (occurring within days of head injury) and chronic (occurring late in the course, weeks, months, or even years). Some degree of dilation of ventricles is seen in 30–75% of patients with head injury; however, a shunt insertion is required in only 2–6% of patients. In most patients, the hydrocephalus is delayed in onset (the incidence of delayed to acute hydrocephalus is 6 to 1). The most common cause is obstruction to the CSF pathways at the arachnoid villi due to the associated bleeding occurring at the time of injury.

In posttraumatic hydrocephalus, often the intracranial pressure remains persistently elevated, even after the acute phase following the head injury is over. Alternatively, it can manifest as a bulge developing over the surgery site, which is often called a **pseudomeningocele**. A CT scan demonstrates progressive ventricular dilatation, suggesting the diagnosis.

Another common presentation of chronic hydrocephalus is a severely head-injured patient, who fails to maintain improvement, and may slowly deteriorate in cognitive functions while receiving treatment in the rehabilitation facilities. Often, the hydrocephalus can develop quite late, even months or years after the initial trauma. A CT scan of the brain demonstrates progressive enlargement of ventricles. A ventriculoperitoneal shunt, especially a programmable valve (adjustable pressure valve; see later), is commonly considered by most neurosurgeons.

19. What are the other conditions associated with hydrocephalus?

Posthemorrhagic hydrocephalus: In subarachnoid hemorrhage (SAH), commonly caused by a ruptured aneurysm, spontaneous bleeding occurs in the subarachnoid spaces and

Pseudomeningocele

An abnormal collection of cerebrospinal fluid (CSF) communicating with the normal CSF surrounding the brain or spinal cord.

Posthemorrhagic hydrocephalus

Hydrocephalus resulting after bleeding inside the brain with the blood products obstructing the cerebrospinal fluid pathways.

the surface of the brain. Most often there is associated bleeding into the ventricles. Blood can obstruct the CSF pathway either in the subarachnoid space or in the ventricles, resulting in hydrocephalus. Approximately 25–30% of SAH patients develop acute hydrocephalus. Acute hydrocephalus is usually treated by an external ventricular drain (a tube placed to drain the bloody CSF to a collection bag under sterile conditions). If the blockage continues, it requires placing a ventricular shunt.

Following subarachnoid hemorrhage, ventricles can dilate slowly over weeks. Dilatation of the ventricles produces plateauing of the improvement or progressive neurologic deterioration. The placement of a shunt from either the ventricles or the lumbar spinal region is usually considered. Sometimes, serial lumbar punctures can be useful and a shunt placement can be avoided.

Normal pressure hydrocephalus: Normal pressure hydrocelphalus is common in older populations and has special considerations; therefore, we will discuss it later in detail. However, it is a type of communicating hydrocephalus with open CSF pathways within the ventricles. The obstruction is commonly considered to be at the level of the arachnoid villi. These patients are usually older and present with a classic triad of gait ataxia, dementia (memory impairment), and urinary urgency and incontinence. They usually benefit from ventriculoperitoneal shunt insertion with sometimes remarkable improvement.

Hydrocephalus associated with achondroplasia: Achondroplasia is characterized by dwarfism and is associated with decreased longitudinal growth of the proximal bones of the body with diminished growth of the base of the skull. About 11% of patients with achondroplasia will have significant hydrocephalus to require a shunt. In achondroplasia, stenosis of several skull base foramina leads to obstruction of the venous flow out of the brain, thus causing raised venous pressure. Slow absorption of the CSF results, causing communicating hydrocephalus. It commonly presents as large head (macrocrania). CT and MRI scans show enlarged subarachnoid spaces, widened sulci, and mild to moderate ventricular enlargement. CT angiography or MR venography can often demonstrate stenosis of jugular foramen.

In view of the communicating hydrocephalus, these patients are ideally treated by ventriculoperitoneal shunt insertion. The overall prognosis related to the hydrocephalus is usually good.

PART SIX

Radiological Picture of Hydrocephalus

How does the MRI scan improve the diagnosis of hydrocephalus?

Is MRI required in all patients with hydrocephalus?

What is a shunt series? When does it need to be done?

More...

20. What is a CT scan? Can you make me understand what my doctor looks for in the CT scan?

Let us briefly discuss the principles of CT scan. This will help us better understand hydrocephalus and explain the requirements for follow-up. Computed tomography (or CT scan), developed by the British scientist Sir Godfrey Newbold Hounsfield, was available in early 1970s for clinical use. As we will see later, CT scan is the single most important investigation that has greatly facilitated diagnosing and managing various brain pathologies, including hydrocephalus.

The CT scan essentially slices the head and other parts of the body into multiple sections, with thicknesses varying from 1 millimeter to 10 millimeters. Normally, 5-millimeter sections are used for the CT scan of the head. These slices are then individually viewed. In simple terms, it is like slicing a loaf of bread into multiple slices and viewing the slices individually. The new-generation CT scans can reconstruct slices to show a three-dimensional picture.

Now, let us go through the CT scan of a normal individual (**Figure 10 to Figure 13**). Notice that some areas in the CT scan appear white, some appear gray, and some are dark. Conventionally, most structures viewed in a CT scan are compared with adjacent brain structures. The normal brain appears gray. The CT scan essentially measures the density of the brain structures and plots them across a gray scale. The more compact or dense structures appear more white (hyperdense), whereas the less dense structure appears darker (hypodense). The density of the structure in the CT scan is measured in a unit called the Hounsfield unit (HU). Hence, the most compact bone is the whitest, and air, which is the least dense, is the darkest. CSF is a mixture of water and some cells, chemicals, and minerals and is, therefore, slightly denser than air. CSF appears darker than the adjacent brain but less dark than the air. In Figure 10, we can see that there is a white rim encompassing the gray structures. This white rim is the skull bone (compare it with the crust of the bread), the relatively dark areas in the center are the CSF, and the adjacent gray areas are the brain tissue. The brain has two types of tissue, gray matter and white matter. Gray matter is slightly more compact and has a slightly more whitish appearance than white matter. This difference may not always be apparent and is often picked up only by an experienced eye. Although they are intermingled, gray matter predominates in the surface (underneath the bone), while white matter is more toward the central part of the brain. Notice that the structure outside the white rim of bone, which is the atmospheric air (surrounding our skull) is quite dark.

Next, we will discuss the orientation in the CT scan. With the CT scan, we view the slice from the lower end of the body. Hence, the left side of the brain is represented on the right side of the image. This pattern is followed by most of the CT scanners available today, though an occasional CT scan views the brain in the reverse. The side of the body is represented in each slice on its sides as R or L, indicating whether it is the right or left side of the body. Hence, it is important for us to identify the correct side in the CT scan image. Some surgeries done on the wrong side can be traced to not remembering this aspect of the CT scan images. Fortunately, the orientation of the front and back match the patient's actual head position: The front of the image represents the front of the patient.

As we discussed earlier, bone is hyperdense (whiter) and CSF is hypodense (darker) as compared with brain tissue. Density measurements are used to predict consistency of intracranial structures, which often help the physician to arrive at a diagnosis. Clotted blood is hyperdense as compared with liquefied blood, which is isodense or hypodense. Calcification (formation of abnormal bone) also appears hyperdense. Hypodense structures include CSF, pus, and fat. To summarize, density in descending order follows: bone, calcification, clotted blood, brain tissue, CSF, fat, and air. Further, to identify problems, we need to conceptualize the three-dimensional image of the brain and ventricles. It may be slightly difficult initially, but with practice one can do it. Slices are usually arranged from bottom to top and stacked up to constitute the complete cranium.

Contrast-injected scans are often performed to see whether any portion of the brain enhances. Enhancement (becoming denser or whiter in the scans) indicates breakage or disruption of the blood-brain barrier in those regions. Contrast injection usually occurs in most tumors, infections, abscesses, and vascular structures (the contrast-injected through the veins lights up the abnormal blood vessels). It is also seen in conditions and processes in which new tissue forms (granulation tissue). Its role in assessing hydrocephalus is limited to diagnosing any abnormal mass lesion that blocks the pathway, resulting in hydrocephalus.

Let's take some representative CT slices and evaluate them individually.

Slice 1 (Lower slice) (Figure 10): In this section, the eyeball (E) and often the optic nerve (responsible for vision), the nasal prominence in between the eye balls, the right and left ear lobes and the back of the head can be well identified. As we can conceptualize, this section goes through the base of the skull as evidenced by the eyes, ear lobes, and the relatively thick skull bones. The area of the brain behind the bone prominences is the posterior fossa, which includes the cerebellum (C) and the brain stem (BS). The fourth ventricle (FV) can be seen as a small slit.

Slice 2 (intermediate slice-1) (Figure 11): In the intermediate slices (through the forehead), the eyeballs are no longer seen, the ventricles appear more prominent, and the lateral (LV) and third ventricles (TV) are well seen. The part of the brain on both sides of the third ventricle is the hypothalamus–thalamus (T) is complex and consists of very tightly packed dense brain tissue.

Contrast-injected CT scan

This indicates that the CT scan was performed with injecting contrast (a radiographic dye that is easy to visualize in the CT scan). Contrast-enhanced CT scan is usually necessary for diagnosing tumors, infections, and blood vessel abnormalities.

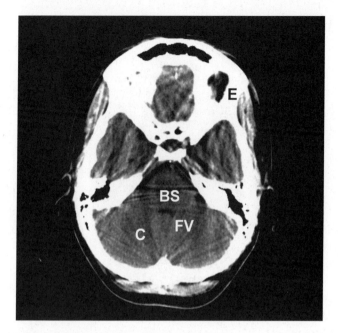

Figure 10.   Normal CT Scan: Fourth Ventricle.

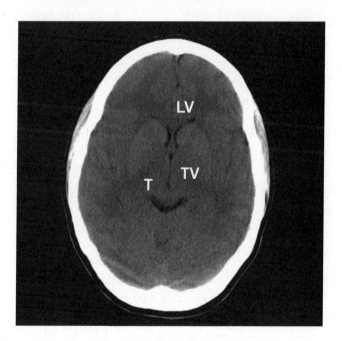

Figure 11.   Normal CT Scan: Third Ventricle.

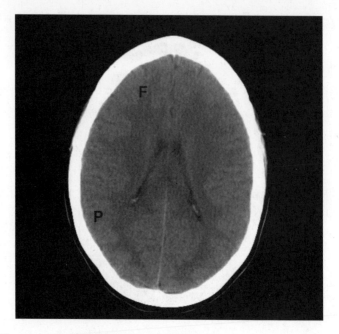

Figure 12. Normal CT Scan: Lateral Ventricle.

Slice 3 (intermediate slice-2) (Figure 12): In this slice, the body of the lateral ventricle is well seen. The frontal (F) and parietal (P) lobes are also well seen. Usually, in patients with hydrocephalus with a shunt surgery, the shunt tube also can be seen in these slices.

Slice 4 (top slice): The ventricles are faintly or no longer seen. The brain matter fills up the cranial cavity, and the parietal lobes are well seen in these slices. The cranial size reduces in the slice as the section goes though the cranial vault.

21. What do I look for in the CT scan in hydrocephalus?

CT scans are the most common investigations ordered in a patient with hydrocephalus. This is because they are fast, available in emergency rooms of even small hospitals, and provide a reasonable amount of information. A CT scan takes approximately less than 5 minutes to perform. The CT scan gives adequate information regarding the existence of hydrocephalus, the degree of hydrocephalus, the type of hydrocephalus, and the possible etiology (cause) of hydrocephalus.

As mentioned earlier, hydrocephalus indicates an accumulation of excessive CSF in the ventricles or in the subarachnoid spaces. As the CSF is less dense than the brain, it is relatively dark in the CT scan. Any excess accumulation can be picked up easily in the CT scans. Normally, the lateral ventricles are small (Figure 12), the third ventricles are barely visible (Figure 11), and the temporal horns are not well seen. In hydrocephalus, depending on the location of the obstruction, either one or all of the ventricles can dilate (**Figure 13**). Dilatation of one ventricle (**unilateral hydrocephalus**) or both ventricles (**biventricular hydrocephalus**) results due to obstruction of one or both foramina of Monro. Obstruction at the level of the aqueduct causes dilatation of the third ventricles in addition to the lateral ventricles (**triventricular hydrocephalus**).

Unilateral hydrocephalus

Dilatation of one lateral ventricle results in unilateral hydrocephalus. The common cause in obstruction at one of the foramen of Monro.

Biventricular hydrocephalus

Dilation of both lateral ventricles results in biventricular hydrocephalus.

Triventricular hydrocephalus

Commonly resulting from aqueductal obstruction, triventricular hydrocephalus results in dilatation of the two laterals and the third ventricle.

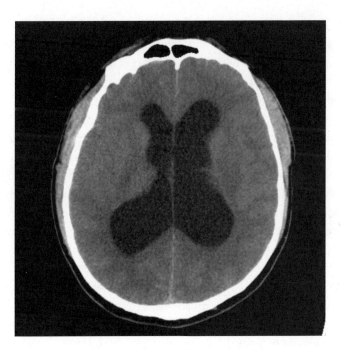

Figure 13. CT Scan in Hydrocephalus. Note the dilated ventricles.

The fourth ventricle along with the other ventricles dilates in obstruction at the level of foramen of Magendie and Luschka (**fourth ventricular outlet obstruction**). In patients with **communicating hydrocephalus**, all ventricles are moderately dilated along with having prominent subarachnoid spaces and basal cisterns.

Types of hydrocephalus: The segment of the ventricles prior (proximal) to the obstruction dilates, whereas beyond (distal to) the obstruction, pathways are not visualized well. This can be well conceptualized when one compares the ventricles to the canals or channels used for drainage. As all the ventricles are usually well visualized in the CT scan, the CT scan can reasonably well indicate the level of obstruction. Most tumorous pathology also can be well visualized in the CT scan. However, the CT scan cannot delineate the exact nature or site of the obstruction. An MRI scan is useful in these circumstances.

CT scan in shunt malfunctions: Probably the greatest utility of the CT scan in managing hydrocephalus has been in assessing patients with shunts with possible malfunction. An obstructed shunt commonly, *though not always*, leads to dilatation of the ventricles, which can be easily diagnosed in the CT scan. In addition, the radio-opaque shunt tube is well seen in the CT scan. The CT scanogram also demonstrates the shunt tube in the upper part of the neck, thus identifying any disconnection in the tube. Because each patient is different, and because the brains of each patient behave differently to the drainage of CSF, comparing previous CT scans is essential. As we will discuss in later chapters, most neurosurgeons would like to compare a CT scan with one done when the shunt was functioning well and the patient was asymptomatic. This is usually performed approximately 6 to 8 weeks after the shunt revision, which is why most pediatric neurosurgeons would like to have a CT done approximately 6 to 8 weeks after placement of a shunt or a revision of the shunt.

Communicating hydrocephalus

(Also known as nonobstructive hydrocephalus) Indicates that the cerebrospinal fluid is in free communication between the ventricular system and the subarachnoid spaces.

22. How does the MRI scan improve the diagnosis of hydrocephalus?

The ability of MRI to obtain images in three different planes (coronal: front to back, sagittal: side to side, and axial: bottom to top) has been considerably valuable in diagnosing the exact cause of hydrocephalus and obstruction in the CSF pathway. As we discussed earlier, the CT scan can indicate the site of the obstruction indirectly (i.e., usually the obstruction cannot be visualized but inferred, depending on the ventricles dilated and the overall pattern). However, with a properly acquired MRI, the site of obstruction often can be well visualized in patients with obstructive hydrocephalus. This is important because small tumors or cysts can be visualized, which, when removed, can relieve hydrocephalus. Later, we will see that MRI is essential to considering endoscopic third ventriculostomy or aqueductoplasty, which are shunt-free alternatives in managing hydrocephalus. Also, MRI assesses the effectiveness of endoscopic third ventriculostomy during the follow-up.

Basic principle of MRI: The principle of the MRI is complex and outside the scope of this book. In extremely simple terms, MRI uses high-powered magnetic field to get a response from the small "biologic magnets," which are basically protons (nucleus of the hydrogen atom). Protons are randomly distributed in the body under normal circumstances. With the patient inside the MRI scanner, initially a high-powered magnetic field (approximately 30,000 times stronger than the earth's magnetic field) is delivered to these protons, which in turn align themselves to the magnetic field. These protons are then exposed to a strong beam of radio waves. This spins the various protons of the body and the faint signal produced is detected by the receiver of the MRI. The transmitted signal is then processed by a computer and used to construct internal images of the body structure, which is then viewed with a monitor. As in the CT scan, sometimes a contrast injection is given to identify areas taking up the contrast. Normally, contrast stays localized within the blood vessels and does not enter the adjacent brain. However, in patients with abnormal brain structures (e.g., tumors, stroke), it can dissipate, and the adjacent structure looks whiter in certain images. Contrast enhancement is usually performed if a tumorous, infectious, or vascular pathology is suspected.

Interpretation of the MRI in a patient with hydrocephalus: The greatest advantage of the MRI is that it can section the brain in three different planes. In addition, the MRI scan is versatile, as it can acquire several types of images, depending on the duration of the stimulus and its time of acquisition. Normally, in a MRI scan, one can see several sequences of images. We will discuss some common sequences, as images of the same slice can appear strikingly different in different sequences. The most common ones are T1 weighted images (also known as T1), T2 weighted images (called T2), and FLAIR images. Sometimes neurosurgeons order specific sequences for hydrocephalus, which are usually fiesta or CISS 3D and CSF flow studies (cine flow images). Many sequences can be performed by varying the duration of stimulus and the time duration until when the signals are acquired. Three planes of image sectioning are axial (top to bottom), sagittal (side to side), and coronal (front to back).

Sagittal MRI (Figure 14): The midsagittal images are the most important images in the MRI scan of a patient with hydrocephalus. These images reveal lateral (LV), third (TV), and fourth (FV) ventricles and the aqueductal region (AQ). The foramen of Monro is best seen in the images just to the right and left of the midsagittal image. The most useful information gained in the midsagittal image is the region of the aqueduct and the third ventricular floor. As the conventional MRI images are 5-millimeter slices, the fine details of the aqueductal anatomy and the pathology may be missed in routine imaging sequences. In this regard, most neurosurgeons will request thin, overlapping slices in the region of the aqueduct to visualize the abnormality. Some

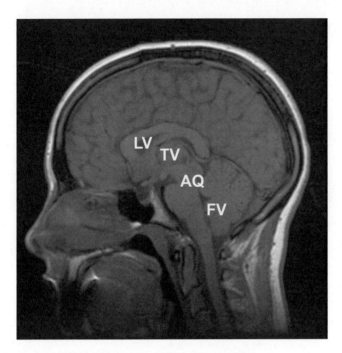

Figure 14.   Normal T1 Weighted Sagittal MRI of Brain.

high-resolution scanners can perform a sequence called as
Fiesta (software devised by General Electric) or CISS 3D
(Siemens), which gives significant details about the anatomy
of the region (Figure 30, p. 121). The status of the third ventricular floor (straight or bulging inferiorly) can indicate the
intrathird ventricular pressure (Figure 30, p. 121). This often
reflects the intraventricular pressure and gives valuable information regarding the severity of the hydrocephalus in relation
to the pressure.

Axial images (Figure 15): The axial images appear similar to
the axial CT scan images although they reveal much more
anatomic distinction between various brain structures than
the CT scan. As we have discussed them in detail in the
CT scan, we will not discuss them further here. The lateral
ventricles (LV), third ventricle (TV), and fourth ventricle are
well seen in the corresponding images.

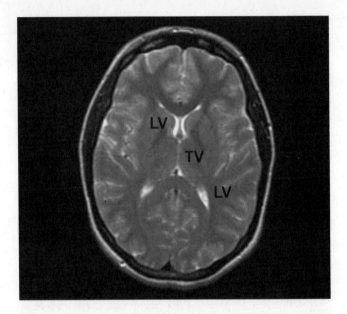

Figure 15. Normal T2 Weighted Axial MRI of Brain.

Coronal images (Figure 16): The coronal images depict lateral ventricles (LV), third ventricle, and the third ventricular floor well. The fourth ventricle and the aqueduct are often not visualized well because of their orientation. The basilar artery and its bifurcation are also well seen.

23. Is MRI required in all patients with hydrocephalus?

This is a pertinent question that many parents and families often ask. This is significant in infants and young children who often have to be sedated or even anesthetized for the MRI. This is concerning because, even though anesthesia is considerably safer today than in the past, occasionally complications arise from the procedure. In addition, a patient has to wait for some time before a MRI can be performed as compared with a CT scan. We will try to discuss the various circumstances in which MRI can be considered essential, desirable, and avoidable under various clinical circumstances associated with hydrocephalus and shunting procedures.

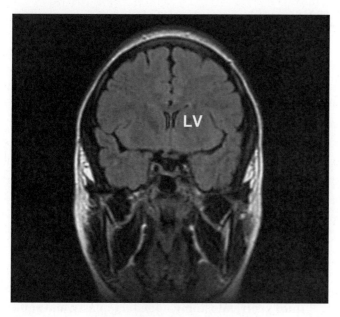

Figure 16. Normal Coronal MRI of Brain (Flair Images).

Situations When MRI Is Considered Essential

1. Patients with newly acquired hydrocephalus when the cause is uncertain

It is essential to rule out an obstructive cause for hydrocephalus before a surgical procedure, such as a shunt insertion, is considered. Unfortunately, some patients with newly diagnosed hydrocephalus who have a small tumor in the region of the aqueduct (tectal glioma) or in the brain stem are diagnosed as obstructive hydrocephalus because of aqueductal stenosis and undergo a shunt insertion with the tumor remaining completely unchecked and undiagnosed till they reach a considerable size. Similarly, a thin-sequence MRI will be able to differentiate between normal pressure hydrocephalus and obstructive hydrocephalus due to aqueductal stenosis. As we will see later, this is important, as patients with aqueductal stenosis can be managed with an endoscopic surgery (endoscopic third ventriculostomy or aqueductal reconstruction procedures), and shunt insertion can be avoided.

Radiological Picture of Hydrocephalus

53

2.   **Patients with brain tumors or other cystic lesions (e.g., arachnoid cyst, cysticercus cysts) causing hydrocephalus**

In clinical practice, it is common to realize that often the obstruction is caused by a cysticercus cyst (a type of brain worm) blocking the narrow CSF pathways at the foramen of Monro or aqueduct. Such occurrences may require direct cyst excision rather than insertion of a shunt for the accompanying hydrocephalus. Arachnoid cysts that cause hydrocephalus are usually in proximity to the ventricular system and often can be communicated with the ventricles by endoscopic procedures avoiding a shunt insertion.

3.   **Patients with hydrocephalus who are candidates for alternative procedures to shunting (endoscopic third ventriculostomy, aqueductoplasty, and aqueductal stenting)**

As we will discuss in later chapters, it is imperative to have MRI in this subgroup of patients to consider the best available surgical procedure.

4.   **Candidates with multiloculated hydrocephalus in whom endoscopic septostomy is considered**

MRI scan often demonstrates the thickness of the septations and the nature of the fluid (proteinaceous, blood stained) that aid in planning the ideal approach and the extent of fenestrations.

Situations When MRI Is Desirable

1.   **Patients who had prior surgery for hydrocephalus and are having multiple shunt malfunctions**

MRI scans often demonstrate additional findings, such as the location of the choroid plexus, which aids in surgical planning or consideration.

Situations When MRI Can Be Avoided

1. Acute shunt malfunctions in previously asymptomatic patients of hydrocephalus with shunt

Usually, acute shunt malfunctions presenting with significant symptoms would not give adequate time for MRI to be performed. If the condition has been diagnosed adequately in the past, a MRI is not indicated before proceeding for shunt revision. If MRI is considered essential, a temporary CSF drainage procedure, such as a shunt tap and release of CSF, exteriorization of the blocked shunt, and CSF drainage or placement of external ventricular drain, is performed. Once adequate CSF is released, an MRI can be considered.

However, it is essential to realize that each patient is different, and generalizations presented have considerable limitations. During my neurosurgical residency, a professor's favorite comment was "Diseases do not read and follow textbooks," which enabled us to realize that every problem has to be approached with an open mind, which is essential for satisfactory outcome.

24. What is a shunt series? When does it need to be done?

A shunt series is a series of X-rays that track the shunt tube through its course (from the head to the site of insertion: peritoneal cavity or the pleural cavity). For this reason, the shunt tubes are intentionally made radio-opaque (they can be identified in the X-rays) by impregnating barium on the tube. This is extremely useful while following up patients with shunts to see whether the tube has fractured, disconnected, or moved from its site of insertion. Usually these take few minutes and can be obtained either in the clinic or the hospital set up. Most neurosurgeons will have it done during the annual follow-up, especially in growing children and adults where the shunt has been in place for few years or more. Shunt series is also useful when the patient has symptoms of shunt malfunction in the emergency setup.

Lata's comment:

Our son Abhi had a shunt placed for his hydrocephalus when he was 2 years old. When he was 12, he started telling us that his head had been hurting. Often he would go to sleep in the afternoon after coming back from school. We did not know why he was having these headaches. When we consulted his neurosurgeon, he obtained a CT scan and a shunt series. The shunt series showed that the shunt was broken in the neck and the lower part had moved into the belly. Our doctor mentioned that this is not uncommon after several years of functioning and that shunts, like other devices, have a "life span." The shunt tube often breaks and the lower part of the tube does not drain the fluid, thus causing the symptoms. We were glad that he picked it up before Abhi further worsened. He replaced the old shunt with a completely new shunt system.

PART SEVEN

Common Bedside Procedures in Hydrocephalus

What is a shunt tap?

What is a ventricular tap?

What is a lumbar drain, and how it is placed?

More...

Several common bedside procedures are often performed in patients with hydrocephalus. We will discuss these procedures briefly in this chapter.

25. What is a shunt tap?

The **shunt tap** is a common procedure performed in patients with ventriculoperitoneal shunt. As we have seen earlier, the shunt tube has a small reservoir (a small bubble), which is designed to use for tapping the shunt. Usually, the shunt taps are performed by neurosurgeons, associates of neurosurgeons (like residents or physician assistants), or sometimes emergency care physicians. Most of the time it is done to diagnose or exclude shunt infection. Sometimes, when in doubt, it is done to assess the functioning of the shunt or to see that if the intracranial pressure is in par with the pressure setting in the shunt.

Most of the time it is done to diagnose or exclude shunt infection.

Usually, the procedure is performed at the bedside or during the clinic visit. It is a minor procedure and does not require any local anesthesia, though in small children who are anxious and frightened, a small dose of sedative may be administered before the procedure. I have found a few minutes of comforting talk and reassurance to work with young children and anxious parents. A thin butterfly needle (also known as the scalp vein, size 23 or thinner) attached to a syringe is introduced through the skin over the shunt tube after the area is prepared and sterilized. Although most neurosurgeons would like to shave a bit of hair off the aspiration site, some may choose to part and clean the area. This is important because infection can be introduced during the tap. It is also possible that aspirated fluid may become contaminated and then yield bacteria in the culture, which often confuses the clinical scenario and may lead to removal of the shunt and reintroduction at a later date. Once the needle is in the reservoir, the CSF may be seen flowing through the tube or can be easily aspirated with a syringe. Both situations indicate a functioning shunt. Fluid is usually clear although it may be mildly pinkish due to minor trauma during the tap. The fluid is collected in several sterile small bottles or tubes and is sent to the laboratory for testing if required. When indicated, the surgeon may connect the other end of the needle to a manometer (used to measure pressure), and the intracranial pressure can be checked. In such cases, it is usually done before aspirating or collecting fluid from the shunt reservoir, as letting out fluid may alter the initial pressure readings.

Sometimes when the shunt tap is performed to assess the shunt's functioning, the surgeon may push back a small amount of fluid into the shunt reservoir to test the patency of the lower end. If the fluid flows easily, the shunt's distal end is considered to be patent, although this observation often can be misleading.

After the procedure, the needle is removed, and the area is inspected for any leaking fluid or oozing blood. Although it is common to find a mild oozing, which usually settles with a small dressing, fluid leakage is uncommon if the appropriate-sized needle is used.

26. What is a ventricular tap?

With a ventricular tap, the needle is passed through the brain tissue and the ventricles are tapped. Although the procedure is classified as a minor procedure, it is slightly more complex and can be associated with significant complications if adequate care is not taken. The procedure is usually limited to neuro-surgeons and their associates who are well versed in anatomy and the procedure's techniques.

To access the ventricles, the skull bones, coverings of the brain (dura, arachnoid, etc.), and brain substance must be traversed. Usually, the latter two structures can be penetrated with a sharp needle, whereas it is impossible to penetrate the skull bone unless it is defective or a hole is made in it. Hence, this procedure is widely used in infants with open fontanels (soft spots) or sometimes in grown-up children and adults with a drill hole made before the tap.

In newborn premature babies, the wide-open fontanel provides easy access to the intracranial compartment. As we have discussed earlier, some premature babies develop intraventricular hemorrhage (IVH), and with the greatest value of this procedure in directly accessing the ventricular compartment, it is widely used in intermittently relieving intracranial pressure and developing hydrocephalus in this population.

Usually, the procedure is performed at the bedside. The proposed tapping site area is cleaned and thoroughly prepared to ensure sterility. The lateral edges of the anterior fontanel (soft spot, felt just above the forehead) on the right side is identified. The left side may also be used, but the right side is preferred as it is usually the nondominant brain in most of the population. Usually, the extreme lateral-most point is chosen to enter the intracranial cavity because the farther away from midline, the less the likelihood of injury to the sagittal sinus (the midline large venous channel) or the veins draining to it (the cortical veins converge toward the midline as they enter the sagittal sinus). The intracranial cavity is entered with a 23-gauge butterfly, and the needle is advanced for about 2–2.5 centimeters (1 inch). The angle of the entry is important. It should be perpendicular to the scalp and the bone to traverse the least distance. If the ventricles are large, then the needle tip usually is in the ventricle and fluid can drain or gently aspirate. During aspiration, carefully and slowly release the fluid, as a sudden drop in intracranial pressure can cause headache or intraventricular hemorrhage. The amount of fluid removed varies, depending on the indication as a diagnostic procedure or as a therapeutic measure.

Possible complications include introducing infection (very low risk), intraventricular bleeding (low risk), brain injury (very low risk, but possible as the needle traverses through the brain), developing bleeding in the subdural space (uncommon, but possible if the needle injures a vein), or seizures. In patients requiring repeated ventricular taps, a track (or "puncture porencephaly") is often visualized in the CT or MRI scans, indicating frequent passage through the same path. Its overall clinical significance is not very well known.

27. What is a reservoir tap?

Tapping a subcutaneous ventricular reservoir is often used in patients who require repeated ventricular tapping for a length of time (most commonly in premature children with intraventricular hemorrhage requiring frequent ventricular taps). The advantage of the procedure is its easy access and the nonrequirement of the transcerebral passage of the needle every time the tap is done. It reduces such complications as intraventricular hemorrhage, subdural hemorrhage, or brain injury. However, the risk of infection remains. The procedure is easy and similar to a shunt tap. It requires a surgical procedure to implant the reservoir in the subcutaneous plane, so some of the benefits may be offset by the associated surgical procedural risk, which, however, remains low.

28. What does my doctor mean by placing an external ventricular drain?

Placing an external ventricular drain is often considered in patients who are shunting dependent and require a temporary alternative measure of CSF drainage. Examples of indications include management of shunt infection, temporarily relieving high intracranial pressure in an emergency situation (associated with shunt malfunction, in subarachnoid hemorrhage), when hydrocephalus is considered reversible (hydrocephalus associated with brain tumors in which hydrocephalus often resolves after tumor surgery), or when hydrocephalus is associated with bleeding in the ventricles (intraventricular hemorrhage).

Usually, the procedure is performed either in the intensive care unit or in the operating room by neurosurgeons or trained associates. The area needs to be shaved and prepared. If the patient has a previous entry site (like with an indwelling shunt), then the same burr hole site is used. If not, either a drill hole (usually if it is in intensive care unit) or a burr hole (if performed in the operating room) is done. The advantages of a burr hole are that it gives a relatively larger area for access and has a slightly lesser chance of subdural or epidural bleeding. However, for the burr hole, the patient is usually transferred to the operating room and the procedure is performed under general anesthetics. As there is usually a time lag, in an emergency, placing the external drain by a drill hole is favored. Sometimes in premature or newborn infants the catheter can be passed through the open fontanel with a special needle. After access to the intracranial compartment is made and the dural covering is opened, a catheter mounted on a stilette or a ventricular tap needle is passed through the brain at a suitable angle to reach the ventricles. The CSF usually is seen dripping out from the open end of the catheter or the needle. After a few milliliters of CSF is collected, the catheter is tunneled under the skin for a certain length (to prevent infection), brought out through a separate opening, and then secured in position. Sometimes the surgeon makes several loops of catheter on the skin surface and then fixes them to prevent accidental dislodgement. The catheter is then connected to a closed drainage system, which is then kept at a required height to drain the fluid.

29. Please tell me something about routine care of the external drain after it is placed.

The external ventricular drainage system is a closed system, thus minimizing the risk of infection. However, as the catheter communicates from the intracranial compartment to the outside, there is a possibility of infection. Usually, infection travels from the skin surface to the ventricle through the catheter. The risk of infection usually increases significantly after the seventh day. However, often infection can be avoided by following careful measures as outlined:

a. Keep the drain insertion site dry, clean, and covered with a sterile dressing.

b. Change the dressing and clean the insertion site at least once every 3 days.

c. Most neurosurgeons send CSF for evaluation once in every 2 days to look for any signs of infection before it is clinically apparent. However, some argue that this is not cost-effective, and CSF needs to be sent only when an infection is strongly suspected or diagnosed.

d. Prophylactic antibiotics: This is a controversial topic and several recent studies have shown that administration of prophylactic antibiotics does not actually reduce the chance of infection. However, the patient is often on antibiotics if there is evidence of infection elsewhere in the body or if the drain is placed for shunt infection.

Most of the time, the issue requiring the placement of the drain clears within a week's time and the drain is removed or replaced with a shunt procedure. However, often the drain is still required, and in such cases, most neurosurgeons replace it with another drain in another exit point in the skin, although the same burr hole site is used. Some, however, would still continue to use the same drain system with extra caution to look for any early signs of infection.

The drainage bag is often set at a height of 10–15 centimeters initially, though this varies significantly from case to case and with the indication for drain placement. For instance, in patients with gross intraventricular hemorrhage, it is often desired to keep the drain at a height of 5–10 centimeters until the blood resolves. However, during later stages, the drain is usually elevated to a height of 20 or 25 centimeters to assess the brain's tolerance to adapt to the increased fluid retained by the elevated drain. The drainage catheter is often connected to an intracranial pressure monitoring system, which monitors the intracranial pressure to ascertain whether the patient is developing any increased intracranial pressure.

While the drain is in place, the nurse usually monitors hourly and daily output from the drain. This is important because it indicates how much fluid should be diverted out by the drain. This indirectly indicates the amount of CSF absorbed by the body. As we have discussed, approximately 500 milliliters (16 ounces) of CSF is produced by choroid plexus every day. Drainage of a relatively large amount of fluid (e.g., 300 milliliters) indicates that the brain's own absorption system is not absorbing the fluid adequately, suggesting a shunt or permanent CSF diversion procedure is required.

Weaning off from the drain: Your doctor will likely want to wean you off the drain. During weaning, the drain is progressively elevated to a higher level and then clamped, while the intracranial pressure and the clinical condition are monitored closely. Most doctors will perform a CT scan intermittently to assess any increase in ventricular size. Weaning often requires a few days of observation, during which it's decided whether the drain needs to be replaced with a permanent shunt device. Indications for continued CSF drainage include clinical deterioration (drowsiness, worsening headache), raised intracranial pressure, or enlarged ventricular size in the CT scans. With any of these, either alone or in combination, a decision to perform a permanent CSF diversion procedure is made. Your neurosurgeon would be the ideal person to arrive at the decision.

30. What is a lumbar drain, and how it is placed?

Often it is desirable to drain the CSF from the lumbar spinal space rather than from the ventricular space. In such cases, a lumbar drain is placed. The procedure is usually done at the bedside and is similar to a spinal tap. The patient is positioned in the lateral position, and after local anesthesia, the spinal tap is performed using a slightly thicker needle. After CSF is obtained, the thin lumbar drain catheter is guided into the lumbar spinal space through the needle. The needle is removed, and the catheter is tunneled in the subcutaneous space and brought out and connected to the fluid collection system. The lumbar drain bag is adjusted at the desired level. Care and further management of the lumbar drain is similar to ventricular drain management.

PART EIGHT

Indications for Surgery for Hydrocephalus

What are the different surgical options for hydrocephalus?

Does everyone with a dilated ventricle need surgery?

My son has hydrocephalus. Can he be managed medically?

More...

31. What are the different surgical options for hydrocephalus?

Surgery for hydrocephalus involves diversion of the accumulated CSF either (a) by reopening the obstructed normal pathways, (b) by creating a diversion before the obstruction so that the CSF drains into the intracranial pathways distal to the block, or (c) by diverting the CSF into another cavity. Examples of reopening of the obstructed pathway include endoscopic aqueductoplasty and excising the tumor that causes hydrocephalus. Endoscopic third ventriculostomy falls into the second category. Ventriculoperitoneal shunts belong to the third group.

Although shunts have been the mainstay of treatment, endoscopic procedures have been recently considered in a selected group of patients. These include endoscopic third ventriculostomy, endoscopic aqueductoplasty, and endoscopic aqueductal stenting. These procedures, though exciting, require strict patient selection criteria and are only indicated in specific circumstances. We will discuss these options in detail later.

32. Does everyone with a dilated ventricle need surgery?

It is often difficult for the pediatric neurosurgeon to decide whether the patient with ventriculomegaly needs a cerebrospinal fluid diversion procedure. In children or adults with enlarging ventricles and symptoms of raised intracranial pressure, the decision is straightforward. However, as we discussed in earlier chapters, the decision for inserting a shunt in older children or adults with minimal symptoms and ventriculomegaly is difficult. Imaging studies and invasive procedures, such as intracranial pressure monitoring, do not reliably predict which patients are likely to develop intellectual deterioration as a result of hydrocephalus.

The ultimate goal in treating hydrocephalus is reversing the neurologic damage caused by the raised intracranial pressure.

Reconstituting the cerebral mantle (the thickness of the cortex of brain) to allow normal intellectual development and avoiding shunt dependency should be considered additional goals in managing hydrocephalus. In one study, cerebral mantle thickness of 2.7 centimeters or more was found to be associated with good outcome. It was also found that cortical mantle reconstitution was not satisfactory if the treatment was delayed for more than 5 months.

It is suggested that children younger than 5 years of age with moderate or severe hydrocephalus without any symptoms are preferably treated with a CSF diversion procedure, as it is often difficult to assess the intellectual development in this age group. Mere attainment of developmental milestones does not indicate adequate development of intellectual function. Inserting a CSF shunt protects these children against a future "damaging" effect of persistent ventriculomegaly and ascertains optimal environment for future intellectual development. However, children older than 5 years and adults with asymptomatic ventriculomegaly are often closely watched and frequently assessed for intellectual development before a shunt insertion is considered.

33. How is hydrocephalus managed under these circumstances?

a. **Myelomeningocele and hydrocephalus:** Approximately 80% of children with myelomeningocele will require treatment for associated hydrocephalus. The timing of insertion of the ventriculoperitoneal (VP) shunt varies from center to center. Simultaneous insertion of the VP shunt and excision of the myelomeningocele has been practiced in the past. Although it shortens the overall hospital stay and reduces the incidence of CSF leak from the wound closure site, this has been associated with an increased incidence of shunt infection and shunt malfunction.

Posterior fossa tumor

Tumors located in the posterior fossa of the cranial cavity. The common tumors located in posterior fossa are medulloblastoma, ependymoma, cerebellar glioma, and intracranial metastatic tumors. These tumors commonly cause hydrocephalus by obstructing the cerebrospinal fluid pathways.

Posttraumatic ventriculomegaly

Dilatation of the ventricles following significant brain trauma. The excessive cerebrospinal fluid accumulation does not usually require a surgical intervention.

b. **Posterior fossa tumor and hydrocephalus:** Hydrocephalus associated with posterior fossa tumor may require a shunting in the preoperative period. Routine preoperative shunting is currently not practiced, and most patients can be managed by external ventricular drain placement or a third ventriculostomy and establishing CSF pathways at surgery. A subtotal tumor removal or a persistent hydrocephalus in the postoperative period would warrant a shunt placement.

Lee et al. (1994) studied 42 children with posterior fossa tumor and hydrocephalus who were not shunted either before or immediately after surgery. Of these, 40% required shunts as late as 4 weeks into the postoperative period. This study indicated that more than half of the patients did not require a shunt insertion either in the immediate or in the late postoperative period (Lee et al., 1994).

c. **Posttraumatic ventriculomegaly:** Dilated ventricles after a severe head injury often can be interpreted either as hydrocephalus or as atrophy and compensatory ventriculomegaly. Often, these patients are in rehabilitation facilities and have either a slow improvement or a plateau in neurologic recovery. These cases challenge the neurosurgeon to decide whether the patient would benefit from a shunt insertion. Most neurosurgeons consider placing a shunt if a slow deterioration is associated with dilated ventricles. However, in the absence of deterioration, transient improvement after a spinal tap and large volume CSF drainage may be helpful in considering placing a shunt. Some neurosurgeons may consider a close follow-up and intermittent CT scans to assess ventricular dilatation, which may indicate placing a shunt.

34. My son has hydrocephalus. Can he be managed medically?

Frankly speaking, medical management has not proved useful in hydrocephalus. It is often used as a temporary measure and in conjunction with surgical management. The most commonly used drug is Diamox (acetazolamide), which has been found to reduce CSF production to a certain extent. However, benefits are minimal, and the drug must be given in high doses to be effective; however, with high doses, side effects are common.

PART NINE

Shunts: The Basics

What are shunts? Can you let me know more about the components of the shunt system?

What are the various types of shunt?

What is siphoning? How it can be prevented?

More...

To keep shunts functioning forever has remained an enigma. Although the concept of shunt appeared to be simple, it has proved to be complex. Of course, the brain is a complex organ, and hydrocephalus is a dynamic process that cannot be simply cured by inserting a mechanical device such as a shunt. We will discuss some important concepts and principles about shunts, which will help us later in management.

35. What are shunts? Can you tell me more about the components of the shunt system?

CSF shunts are tubes with valves that drain the CSF out from one compartment to another. One of the first shunts was the ventriculojugular shunt (from the ventricles to the jugular vein in the neck) placed by Nulsen and Spitz in 1952. In 1955, John Holter developed a silicone shunt with slit valves, which was probably the forerunner of present-day shunts. There have been several modifications and additions to this initial concept.

The shunt contains three parts: (1) the ventricular end, (2) the valve complex, and (3) the distal end (**Figure 17**). The distal end is usually named for the organ in which it is inserted (e.g., in ventriculoperitoneal shunts, it is known as the peritoneal end; in ventriculoatrial shunts, the atrial end).

Ventricular catheter

The part of the shunt catheter that enters the ventricles. This connects to the valve complex.

Ventricular catheter: The ventricular end has several holes at the tip that let the CSF drain out from the ventricles. The holes are normally circumferentially placed and extend for a length of 1–2 centimeters from the tip. At times, flanges are added to it. Some other shunts have slots with holes. Usually, the tip is a closed end (unless the catheter is a special type used for endoscopic shunt placement). The catheter is trimmed to an appropriate length by the neurosurgeon before the surgery. Some neurosurgeons favor a right-angled sleeve placed around the catheter, usually at the point it exits from the skull. Most ventricular catheters are introduced from either the frontal (behind the hairline) or the parietal

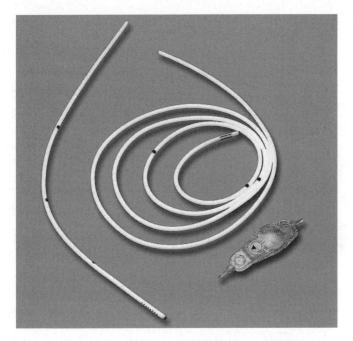

Figure 17. Photograph of a Commonly Used Ventriculopritoneal Shunt (Proximal Catheter, Valve with Integrated Antisiphon Device, and Distal Tube).

Courtesy of Medtronics

(behind and above the ear) approach. However, sometimes the neurosurgeon decides the ideal place to insert per the ventricular dilatation. Usually, there are two diameters of ventricular catheters: regular diameter and thinner diameter. Thinner diameters of the catheters are often preferred in neonates and younger children.

The valve complex: This is the most important part of the shunt tube. It can be a simple or complex unit and vary in each type of shunt. As we will see later, there are several types of valves that essentially regulate the flow of CSF through the tube. Most valves have a built-in reservoir, which is basically a small bubble placed proximally to the valve containing CSF (Figure 17 and **Figure 18**). It is used to aspirate fluid from

Valve complex

The valve complex commonly has the reservoir and the valve of the shunt system. At times, the antisiphon device is also integrated with it.

75

CSF Flow

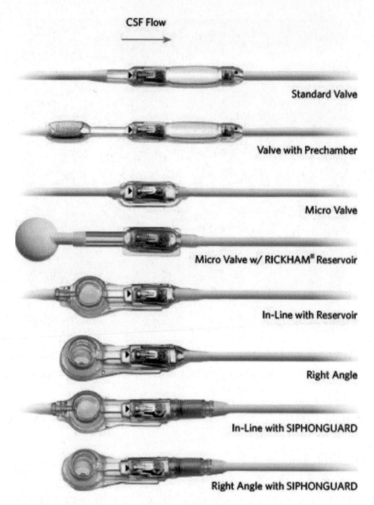

Standard Valve

Valve with Prechamber

Micro Valve

Micro Valve w/ RICKHAM® Reservoir

In-Line with Reservoir

Right Angle

In-Line with SIPHONGUARD

Right Angle with SIPHONGUARD

Figure 18. Various Types of Codman Valves.

Courtesy of Codman, Inc.

the shunt during the shunt tap either to check its patency or to rule out infection. Also after insertion, the patency can be assessed with certain degree of accuracy by compressing it with the pulp of the finger. In most common types of shunts, the reservoir when compressed lets the CSF contained in it flow into the distal tube, thus indicating a distal patency (open distal, e.g., peritoneal end of the tube). Immediately on release of the pressure, the reservoir promptly refills with

CSF sucked in from the ventricles, which indicates proximal patency (patent ventricular end of the tube). Hence, a reservoir that empties well and refills briskly suggests a patent distal end and a patent ventricular end, indicating a patent shunt tube. In the same context, a shunt reservoir that empties well and does not refill (or is collapsed and does not refill) indicates a blocked proximal end. However, a nonemptying full reservoir indicates a nonfunctioning or blocked distal end. A patent shunt tube does not indicate that the shunt is functioning appropriately, as the valves can malfunction by not keeping up to the specifications. In addition, some shunt reservoirs have an incompetent proximal end, indicating that the CSF can flow either way at the reservoir's proximal end near its attachment to the ventricular catheter. This can be misinterpreted as a functioning shunt, as the CSF flows between the reservoir and the ventricles and not through the distal end. In obese individuals or in the immediate postoperative period, it may be difficult to feel the reservoir. In some types of shunts, the reservoir is placed at the burr hole site (burr hole type of reservoir) (**Figure 19**).

Antisiphon devices: These are small devices that prevent siphoning of the CSF that can result in overdrainage when the person is erect (**Figure 23**). Some shunt valves have built-in antisiphon devices placed distal to the valve (Delta Valve, Medtronic), while, in others, the surgeon interposes a stand-alone antisiphon device distal to the valve. As we will discuss later, all patients do not require antisiphon devices. This decision is usually made based on the individual patient's requirement.

Antisiphon devices

Small devices interposed in the shunt system to prevent siphoning of the cerebrospinal fluid that often causes overdrainage.

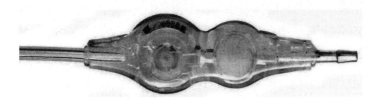

Figure 19. Photograph of Orbis Sigma II Valve (Integra).

Permission granted by Integra LifeSciences Corporation, Plainsboro, NJ.

Distal end: The distal end is a long tube that enters into the draining space, or cavity (Figure 17 and **Figure 24**). When a shunt is introduced into the abdominal cavity (also known as the peritoneal cavity), it is known as the ventriculoperitoneal shunt. Similarly, when a shunt is introduced into the heart (atrium of the heart—entering through the right jugular vein), it is called a ventriculoatrial shunt. The other cavities used are the ventriculopleural or ventriculo-gallbladder shunt.

Some neurosurgeons prefer a single distal tube preconnected to the valve and reservoir (known as **unitized distal end**) because there is less of a chance of disconnection. Often a disconnection occurs at the junction of the valve and distal end. It is also easier to retrieve and remove a shunt with a unitized distal end during subsequent revisions. However, at times, it is preferable to use a nonunitized tube (e.g., interposition of antisiphon device).

The complete length of the shunt tube is nearly radio-opaque (meaning that it can be identified in routine X-rays) because barium impregnates the catheter. The valve is the only part not impregnated with barium, although it has radio-opaque markings to identify the valve type. Evaluating the catheter by X-rays is used during follow-up to identify any disconnected shunt. Some catheters are completely impregnated with barium, while others have a thin strip of barium for radio-opacity.

Most neurosurgeons introduce the entire length of the distal end (usually 90 or 120 centimeters) into the peritoneal cavity. This is particularly beneficial in pediatric patients in which studies have shown that the excess of tube in the abdominal cavity usually accommodates for the required length as the child grows. However, in ventriculoatrial shunts, the lower end is usually limited to the length of the right atrium of the heart.

The terminal end of the distal shunt tube can be either open or closed. Shunts with closed ends have distal slit valves that

Unitized distal end

Here, the valve and reservoir complex of the shunt is unitized with the distal catheter, thus reducing chances of disconnection in the follow-up period.

act as additional valves. Some open terminal ends also have a distal slit valve. Most neurosurgeons prefer to remove the distal slit valves, as studies have revealed a higher chance of lower-end obstruction by omentum (a fibrous fatty structure containing blood vessels present in the abdominal cavity).

Connectors: These can be either straight, right angled, or Y shaped. Straight connectors are used to connect pieces of tube where the right-angled connectors are exclusively used—where the ventricular end connects to the valve. Y connectors are useful to connect one distal tube to two ventricular ends, as in compartmentalized hydrocephalus.

36. What are the various types of shunt?

Shunts can be divided into two broad groups, depending on the types of valves. Commonly, there are two types of valves: (1) differential pressure valves and (2) flow-regulated valves. Differential pressure valves can be fixed pressure valves or variable pressure valves (programmable valves).

Differential pressure valves: These valves open when pressure differs between the CSF pressure and the pressure set in the valve of the shunt (Figure 18). Overall shunt pressure can also be affected by pressure in the receiving cavity (i.e., intra-abdominal pressure), the hydrostatic pressure (which depends on the difference in height between the two compartments, i.e., the cranial and abdominal compartment), and the resistance of the shunt tube.

Under normal circumstances in an adult in a lying down position, pressure in the ventricles is less than 10–15 centimeters of water. It is lower in infants. Pressure falls when an individual is in an erect position; the intracranial pressure is negative. Intra-abdominal pressure is considered equivalent to atmospheric pressure. Conditions that increase pressure of the receiving compartment reduce overall drainage, thus resulting in shunt malfunction. This is sometimes evident in ascites (fluid in

Differential pressure valves

These valves open and close according to a preset opening and closing pressure by the manufacturer. For example, when the intraventricular pressure exceeds the opening pressure, the valve opens and drains the fluid until the pressure drops below the closing pressure, thus stopping the flow.

peritoneal cavity) and chronic constipation in ventriculoperitoneal shunts and pleural effusion in ventriculopleural shunts. When an individual is in an erect position, the difference in height between the upper and lower end of the shunt tube is added to the pressure difference between CSF and shunt valve pressure, thus resulting in increased flow (the principle behind siphoning). In this regard, it can be logically assumed that this effect of siphoning is considerably reduced when an individual is lying down, where the difference in height between the two compartments is almost negligible.

Flow-regulated valve: These incorporate a different philosophy: The CSF is drained out at a constant rate through the shunt valve. The most used flow-controlled valve is the Orbis Sigma Valve, which releases the spinal fluid either at an average of 10 milliliters per hour (low flow valve) or 20 milliliters per hour (Orbis Sigma II) (Figure 19). Although the distal flow may be reduced in conditions that increase receiving compartment pressure (ascites, pleural effusion), the shunt relies less on pressure differences between ventricles and the draining compartment. The greatest advantages of these shunts are that they do not siphon and hence have been found useful in conditions in which siphoning is the predominant concern at follow-up.

Flow-regulated valve
In flow-regulated valve, the cerebrospinal fluid flows at a predetermined constant rate irrespective of the intraventricular pressure. Unlike the differential pressure valves, overdrainage due to siphoning does not occur.

37. What is a programmable valve? Are there special measures required for programmable valves?

Adjustable or programmable shunts: A significant development in the differential pressure valve is the programmable valve, several of which are available now. Normally, a differential pressure valve is manufactured at a set pressure that can vary from very low, low, medium, or high-pressure settings. A low-pressure valve usually has a pressure setting of less than 5 centimeters of CSF pressure with a medium pressure between 5 and 10 centimeters and high pressure between 10 and 15 centimeters of pressure. Once inserted, pressure settings cannot be changed unless a reoperation is done and a new valve is replaced. Intracranial pressure varies significantly between individuals under normal circumstances and in various disease processes. Often after surgery a particular pressure setting is not well tolerated by the individual, and a change is required. The programmable valve is especially useful under such circumstances.

With programmable valves, pressure can be set at one of the various predetermined pressure settings even after the shunt is inserted. A high-powered magnet is used to change the valve settings by placing it over the valve. This is usually an office procedure and takes only few minutes. The available pressure setting varies with the manufacturer, and we will discuss that briefly later. A high magnetic field is used to change the pressure settings; therefore, exposure to a relatively strong magnetic field would change these pressure settings. An MRI scan that uses a high magnetic field changes the pressure setting unless the shunt has a locking mechanism (discussed later). Although widely used home magnets are considered not to alter the pressure settings, a few reports indicate the susceptibility of some programmable valves to relatively lower strength of magnetic fields.

In all the programmable valves, pressure settings are relatively accurate when set appropriately. In some, settings can be confirmed anytime with the device, while in others, the programmer can only confirm the setting immediately after programming the valve. The most commonly used programmable valves are the Hakim programmable valve (Codman), Strata valve (Medtronic), Polaris valve (Sophysa), and the Aesculap-Miethke proGAV valve (Aesculap). As there are some differences between these valves, we will briefly discuss each.

Hakim programmable valve (Codman) (Figure 20): These were the first programmable valves used in the United States and have been in use since the late 1990s when they were first tried in patients with hydrocephalus. The pressure setting varies between 30 and 200 millimeters of CSF pressure (3–20 centimeters of CSF pressure) and can be set at an increment of 10 millimeters of pressure. Thus, it gives a large range of pressure settings that are often beneficial. Valves do not come with a factory preset pressure and hence have to be set before the sterile package is opened in the operating room. The magnetic field during the MRI scan of the brain (or any part of the body) alters the pressure settings, and hence, the valve has to be reprogrammed after the MRI. Pressure settings can be confirmed immediately after programming by the recent version of the programmer (Figure 20), which uses an ultrasound probe during the procedure to count the "number of clicks" that occurs during the reprogramming. However, the earlier version of the programmers lacked this ultrasound probe, and an X-ray confirmation was recommended. The X-ray confirmation is also required if the pressure setting needs to be verified at intervals. X-rays have to be perpendicular

The magnetic field during the MRI scan of the brain (or any part of the body) alters the pressure settings, and hence, the valve has to be reprogrammed after the MRI.

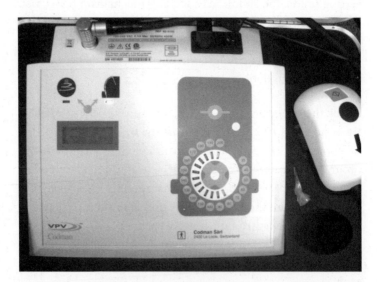

Figure 20. Codman Programming Apparatus. Note the programming levels vary from 30 millimeters of CSF pressure to 200 millimeters of CSF pressure.

Courtesy of Codman, Inc.

to the shunt valve position for an accurate validation, which warrants that the radiographer should have knowledge of the insertion site and valve disposition.

Medtronic Strata valve: The Medtronic Strata valve has five pressure settings (0.5, 1, 1.5, 2, and 2.5), with the 0.5 corresponding to the low range and 2.5 to the high range. The pressure setting of the valve can be checked at any time with the programmer. An MRI scan alters the pressure settings of the shunt. Some strata valves have a built-in antisiphon device (**Figure 21**).

Polaris valve: The Polaris adjustable valve (Sophysa) has the advantage of nonchange of the pressure settings by the MRI scan and other magnetic fields as they happen with Hakim and Strata valves. This is because the valve incorporates a "locking mechanism" in which the valve setting gets locked and cannot be altered unless a reprogramming apparatus is used initially to unlock it.

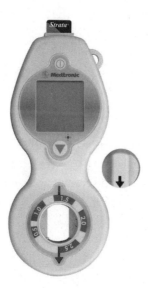

Figure 21. Medtronic Programming Apparatus. Note the programming range varies from 0.5 to 2.5 levels.

Courtesy of Medtronics

Aesculap proGAV programmable valve: The Aesculap-Miethke proGAV programmable shunt system is a titanium-encased, posture-dependent hydrocephalus valve system that is MRI safe for up to 3 Tesla. The unit can be adjusted to a pressure setting between 0 and 20 CSF pressure.

There are many shunt valves in the market that neurosurgeons use. However, it is impossible to describe all of them in this book. Excellent reviews are also available, such as *The Shunt Book* (Drake and Sainte-Rose, 1995).

38. What is siphoning? How it can be prevented?

Siphoning has been considered as a major contributor to overdrainage of CSF. As we have discussed, a shunt diverts fluid from the cranial compartment into another cavity such as the peritoneum, atrium, or pleural cavity. In humans, as we stay erect, the cranial cavity is at a higher elevation than the peritoneal cavity, which causes the CSF to drain through the shunt (siphon) until the fluid level in the absorbing cavity (peritoneal cavity) equilibrates with the level in the ventricular cavity (**Figure 22**). This principle is commonly used in our day-to-day life, such as draining gasoline from a car's gas tank to a container through a tube. However, because it is impossible for the fluid level in the peritoneal cavity to reach the ventricular cavity, the process is almost continuous, causing excess drainage of fluid while an individual is erect. However, lying supine, the cranial and peritoneal cavities are at the same level, siphoning stops, and the shunt drains at its pressure setting. As the atrium is at a higher level than the peritoneal cavity, ventriculoatrial shunts have lower incidence of siphoning as compared with peritoneal shunt. Apart from difference in height, CSF drainage depends on the pressure in the absorbing cavity and compliance of the cranial compartment and the absorbing compartment. Therefore, it is difficult to predict and treat effectively siphoning by antisiphon devices.

Siphoning

In neurosurgical literature, siphoning denotes excessive drainage of cerebrospinal fluid because of difference levels between the ventricles and the distal cavity (e.g., peritoneal cavity, pleural cavity) through the shunt tube.

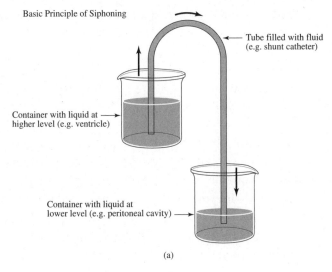

Basic Principle of Siphoning

Tube filled with fluid
(e.g. shunt catheter)

Container with liquid at
higher level (e.g. ventricle)

Container with liquid at
lower level (e.g. peritoneal cavity)

(a)

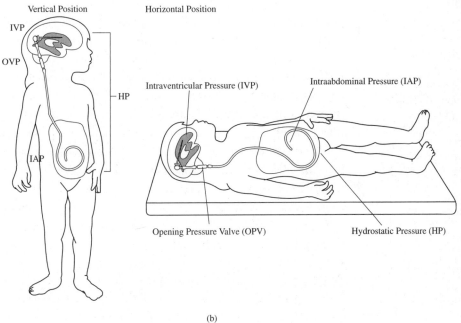

Vertical Position

Horizontal Position

IVP

OVP

HP

Intraventricular Pressure (IVP)

Intraabdominal Pressure (IAP)

IAP

Opening Pressure Valve (OPV)

Hydrostatic Pressure (HP)

(b)

Figure 22. Diagram Showing the Concept Behind Siphoning of CSF.
The difference of height between the ventricles and the peritoneal cavity facilitates siphoning in an upright position.

Adapted from Drake JM and Sainte-Rose C. *The Shunt Book*. Cambridge, MA: Blackwell Science, 1995, page 23.

Shunts: The Basics

There have been several siphon regulatory devices designed to slow down or completely shut off the flow of CSF. Of the several devices available, the most commonly used are the Heyer Schulte antisiphon device (Integra Neurosciences), Delta siphon control device (Medtronic), siphon guard (Codman), and the Shunt Assistant (Aesculap).

The Integra Heyer Schulte antisiphon device incorporates two chambers with a pressure-sensitive membrane in between. Normally, the drainage pathway is open. However, with siphoning, the negative pressure imparts suction on the pressure-sensitive membrane, causing it to close. With developing pressure in the proximal chamber above the atmospheric pressure, the membrane is forced open, causing the CSF to flow. In the siphon control device (Medtronic), the pathway is normally closed and opens when the proximal pressure is higher than the atmospheric pressure. In siphon guard (Codman), the device contains two pathways: (1) a normally open low-resistance pathway and (2) a high-resistance pathway that is normally closed and only opens when the flow exceeds a certain limit (Figure 23). It is justified to assume that the siphon guard functions more as an "antiflow" device than a true antisiphon device. The Shunt Assistant (Aesculap) incorporates a gravitational tantalum ball to reduce flow and comes in various settings of 10, 15, 20, 25, 30, 35, and 40 centimeters of water pressure. Various settings permit wider options to individualize the need for each patient, depending on height and body configuration.

Apart from the previously discussed valves, the Orbis Sigma Valve (IntegraNeurosciences) and the Phoenix Diamond Valve (Vygon Neuro) do not permit siphoning and do not need any additional siphon devices.

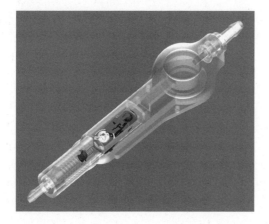

Figure 23. Codman Inline Valve with Integrated Siphonguard.

Courtesy of Codman, Inc.

PART TEN

Shunt Surgery

Can you tell me briefly about shunt surgery? What are alternative sites for inserting the lower end of the shunt?

What are the common complications of shunt surgery?

What are lumboperitoneal shunts?

More...

39. Can you tell me briefly about shunt surgery? What are alternative sites for inserting the lower end of the shunt?

The procedure is usually performed under general anesthesia and takes between an hour and two hours. The patient is placed supine, and the shoulder (of the side where the shunt is being inserted) is slightly elevated with a pillow or a small shoulder roll. The area where the shunt will be placed in the head is shaved and prepared. Some neurosurgeons do not shave but part the hair. The thorax and the abdomen are also prepared. The abdominal shunt insertion site varies from the midline above the umbilicus, right or left upper abdomen, or the paraumbilical region (region of abdomen next the umbilicus) (**Figure 24**). Usually the right side of the cranium and the right abdomen are chosen for shunt insertion. However, the site can be altered, depending on the nature of hydrocephalus and the extent of previous surgery.

Cranial end: Both the parietal and the frontal entry site have been widely used and have their own advantages and disadvantages, with several studies supporting either approach. Conventionally, the ventricular tip of the shunt tube is attempted to be placed away from the choroids plexus in the lateral ventricles, which is why most neurosurgeons have been trained to place it in the frontal horn. Alternatively, some neurosurgeons prefer the atrium of the lateral ventricle because it is the widest part of the ventricle, which is least likely to collapse after the shunt insertion.

Endoscopic guided shunt insertions often use the frontal entry. However, a multicenter trial did not find any difference in the malfunction rate in patients with shunts placed endoscopically compared with the those nonendoscopically placed. Ultrasound guidance is often useful to cannulate small ventricles. Sometimes neuronavigation systems have been used to place the shunt, especially in small ventricles.

Cranial end of the shunt

The part of the shunt entering the intracranial compartment.

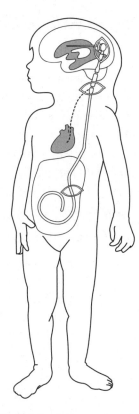

Figure 24. Shunt Insertion Surgery.

Adapted from Netter FH. *The CIBA Collection of Medical Illustrations, Volume I: Nervous System*. CIBA Pharmaceutical Company, 1983, page 9, Section I, Plate 7.

Subcutaneous part: The shunt tube is then tunneled from the cranial incision into the abdominal incision by a thin, long tunneler (shunt passer). This part of the procedure is easy if the catheter is passed in the proper subcutaneous plane.

Distal end: Peritoneal insertion of the distal catheter is most commonly preferred. In the conventional approach, the abdominal cavity is opened by a small incision and the rectus (abdominal) muscles are split. The peritoneum (lining covering the abdominal structures) is opened, and the distal shunt catheter is introduced into the abdominal cavity. Purse string sutures are put in to prevent the tube from slipping out from the abdominal cavity.

Alternatively, in small children, a "peritoneal split trocar" can be used to insert the shunt into the cavity with a very tiny incision. No significant differences have been detected in the outcome by either method. In cases in which the peritoneal insertion is not suitable, the right ventricle or the pleural cavity can be used to insert the distal end.

40. How is the recovery from shunt surgery, and how soon can I take him home?

Recovery from surgery is usually quick. The patient is extubated after the procedure and is conscious in the recovery room. The patient is offered clear liquids few hours after the surgery, and if he tolerates it, his diet is slowly advanced. Most children and adults are discharged the next day. Discharge criteria based on age group need to be fulfilled, which determine the exact discharge day after surgery.

41. What are the common complications of shunt surgery?

Common complications of shunt surgery are malfunction, infection, overdrainage, brain injury, seizures, and distal complications.

42. How does shunt malfunction occur, and how does it present?

Shunt malfunction: Shunt malfunction is the predominant complication of shunt procedures. Malfunction is so common that sometimes it is considered part of the natural history of shunt surgery, rather than as a complication. Of the several predisposing factors for shunt malfunction, age is a significant factor. In the pediatric population, almost one third of shunts fail during the first year of insertion. In a multicenter study involving 38 neurosurgical centers and 773 patients, 29% of shunts failed in the first year, leading to reoperation (Di Rocco, 1994). About half of shunts (47%) inserted in children younger than 6 months of age failed as compared with 14% of shunts that failed in children older than 6 months of age. It was also found that shunts placed as emergency procedures failed more often (34%) than effectively placed shunts (29%).

Obstruction: The most common cause of malfunction is a proximal shunt obstruction, which accounted for 63% of the mechanical complications in the multicenter study. The shunt can be obstructed at several places: at the tip (proximal), at the valve, or at the distal catheter (distal obstruction). The **proximal obstruction** is most commonly due to fronds of choroids plexus or the ependymal or brain tissue blocking the inlet foramina of the ventricular catheter (**Figure 25**). Although placing the shunt in the frontal horn beyond the choroid plexus has the least incidence of blockage, placing the catheter in the most dilated part—the atrium of the ventricle—has also been found to have a lesser incidence of blockage. Occurrence of a slit ventricle has a higher chance of blockage (44%) compared with the normal or mildly enlarged ventricles (27%). This is logical as presence of CSF around the ventricular catheter would prevent its obstruction. For this reason, many neurosurgeons

The most common cause of malfunction is a proximal shunt obstruction

Shunt Surgery

Proximal shunt obstruction

Obstruction of the shunt at the ventricular end. Common obstructive elements are the choroid plexus or brain parenchyma.

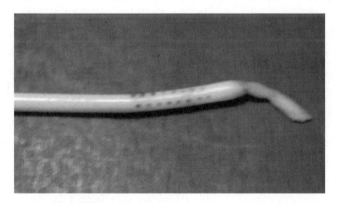

Figure 25. Photogaph of an Obstructed Shunt Catheter with the Holes Near the Tip Blocked by Brain Tissue.

Distal shunt obstruction

Obstruction to the cerebrospinal fluid flow occurring in the distal catheter (e.g., peritoneal catheter in a ventriculoperitoneal shunt).

Ventriculopleural shunt

Shunts draining CSF between the cerebral ventricles and the pleural cavity (pleura is the membrane lining the lungs).

Ventriculoatrial shunts

Shunts draining cerebrospinal fluid between the cerebral ventricles and the atrium (one of the chambers of the heart).

prefer to keep the ventricles slightly large and not completely decompressed or collapsed (slit ventricles). Association of intraventricular hemorrhage during insertion of the shunt is associated with higher incidence of early malfunction.

Distal shunt obstruction in the ventriculoperitoneal shunt is most often due to blockage by omentum (fat in the abdominal cavity). It is also associated with slit valves in the distal end of the closed-ended catheter. These slit valves encourage deposition of debris beneath the slit and cause obstruction. In a previous study, no cases of distal shunt malfunction were found with a distal open catheter while they were associated with presence of distal slit valves.

Loculation of the distal catheter within the peritoneal cavity forms a cyst (pseudoperitoneal cyst), which causes a reduction of drainage of CSF, which causes shunt malfunction. Associated preexisting peritoneal adhesions such as previous surgery or peritonitis can cause loculations. Distal obstruction can also be due to reduced absorption in the abdominal cavity such as chronic infection (tuberculosis), previous surgery, or ascitis (fluid accumulation in the peritoneal cavity).

In cases of **ventriculopleural shunts**, failure of the pleural cavity to absorb fluid leads to symptoms of distal failure and when significant can cause pleural effusion (fluid in the pleural cavity) and cor-pulmonale (cardiac problems due to conditions in the lungs). **Ventriculoatrial shunts** are prone to form thrombi (small blood clots), causing distal obstruction, and can discharge emboli, leading to pulmonary hypertension and renal concerns (shunt nephritis).

Fracture, disconnection, and migration: Shunt components can get disconnected at the junctions and migrate to either cavity. This is more common in the pediatric population, as the growth of the child predisposes the shunt tube to more stress than in the adult population. Limiting the number of connections minimizes the risk of disconnection.

Fracture of the shunt tube, a late complication, is usually observed in a growing child when the shunt is in place for a long time with the ends tethered. Fracture of the shunt tube occurs because silicone degrades and the body reacts to form calcific deposits on the shunt tube. Calcification is more common in the neck and thoracic region than in the abdomen and is extremely uncommon in the ventricular and the abdominal cavities. Fracturing of the tube most often occurs in the neck, with the distal end migrating into the peritoneal cavity (**Figure 26**). The scar tissue track that forms around the tube acts as a CSF conduit for a while, but ultimately fails.

As the scar tissue around the shunt tube forms a conduit and drains the CSF for a while, these patients usually can present

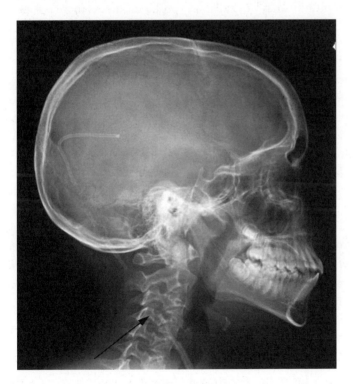

Figure 26. Disconnected Shunt Catheter. Note the discontinuation of the shunt catheter in the neck. (Arrow)

with slow onset of headache. This is unlike the relatively acute or subacute presentation seen in shunt malfunction. However, as the shunt tubes are made radio-opaque, this is easy to diagnose with a "shunt series" X-rays (X-ray of head, neck, chest, and abdomen).

Although it is not difficult, retrieving the disconnected and migrated shunt tube from the subcutaneous tissue and the abdominal cavity is usually not considered because the shunt tube in the subcutaneous tissue may be fragile and break during removal. Some part of the shunt tube distal to the valve may come out during removal along with the valve. The rest of the shunt tube in the subcutaneous tissue is usually left behind as it would require multiple disfiguring skin incisions to remove the degenerated and calcified tube. The left-behind shunt tube may not cause any problems unless there is superadded infection, in which case it is usually removed.

If the distal end of the tube migrates into the abdominal cavity, the tube is left behind (Figure 37, p. 147). It usually freely floats in the abdominal cavity and does not precipitate bowel obstruction. Some neurosurgeons, however, would prefer to remove the abdominal catheter with laparoscopic devices. As in the subcutaneous tissue, the catheter has to be removed if the shunt is.

Sometimes during a shunt revision the ventricular catheter slips inside the track and migrates into the ventricular cavity. In the past, these shunt catheters were left behind; however, with the advent of endoscopic neurosurgery, catheters can be easily grasped and removed with a neuroendoscope. Catheters are removed if the shunt is infected.

43. Please tell me more about shunt infection.

Shunt infection, a nightmare for every neurosurgeon, is the second significant complication after shunt malfunction, which occurs after the tube is inserted. Infection frustrates neurosurgeons who have taken extreme care to insert the shunt and voids the precision with which the shunt was placed.

The current incidence of shunt infection ranges between 4% and 7%. Although few reports indicate a trend toward zero incidence, infection rates of 5–10% are acceptable to most neurosurgical and pediatric neurosurgical centers.

Staphylococcus epidermidis, an organism that commonly resides in the skin, accounts for 40–50% of shunt infections. *Staphylococcus aureus*, another organism, accounts for 20% of shunt infections. *Propionibacterium* species, including diphtheroids, gram-negative bacilli, and *Streptococci* account for 8–10% of the cases. Several risk factors are associated with increased risk of shunt infection. Among these risk factors are prematurity, associated skin infection/disruption, postoperative wound dehiscence, and previous shunt infection appear to be significant, whereas duration of surgery, surgeon's experience, and etiology of the hydrocephalus have been controversial.

Most shunt infections occur within 3 months of insertion. A small percentage occurs as late as 6 months. Most of these organisms normally reside in the skin; therefore, shunt infection probably occurs during insertion. However, these organisms may also reside in the patient's own body because bacteria circulate in the blood and reside on the shunt tube. This is why dentists prescribe antibiotics before dental procedures in patients with indwelling shunt tubes. Some organisms (specifically *Staphylococcus epidermidis*) are known to adhere to the shunt tube and form a biofilm (a slimy layer) that protects bacteria against orally or intravenously administered antibiotics. Usually, bacteria cannot traverse across the shunt tube (from inside to outside or in the reverse direction) unless the shunt tube is broken or disconnected. Colonization permits bacteria to stay quiescent for weeks or sometimes a few months before the infection manifests. This is why neurosurgeons recommend removing the shunt tube completely and reinserting a new shunt tube to manage shunt infections.

Shunt Surgery

Staphylococcus epidermidis

It is one of the bacteria commonly found in skin as a common flora. Although it is usually nonpathogenic, it can cause infection in patients with a compromised immune system.

Organisms that do not form a slimy layer manifest earlier in their presentation.

Clinical picture: A high degree of suspicion for infection in the postoperative period is the key to an early diagnosis. The possibility of a shunt infection should be considered in any patient with a shunt; however, on occasion, only the shunt is related to the fever.

Most shunt infections present within 3 months of insertion, with 90% of these presenting within the first 6 months. This is important as an early infection is only diagnosed with a high degree of suspicion within this period. With decreasing incidence, after 6 months suspicion also decreases.

The clinical picture depends on the severity of the infection, the time of diagnosis, and the site of infection. Shunt infections can be an infection of the shunt tube in its subcutaneous tract or in the wound (wound infection), infection of the CSF spaces or ventricles (ventriculitis, meningitis), or infection of the abdominal space (peritonitis). Early subcutaneous infections present with low low-grade fever, redness along the shunt tube, and purulent discharge from the incision. The wound may break down in some cases with exposure of the tube. Later, as the infection involves the CSF and ventricles, it may be associated with decreased sensorium, seizures, and neurologicalneurologic deficits. If the infection involves the abdominal cavity, it can present with distension, rigidity, and tenderness in the abdominal wall and guarding. Sometimes low-grade infections with *Staphylococcus epidermidis* can present as shunt malfunction.

Diagnosis: Although the diagnosis in the later stages of shunt infection is obvious, the diagnosis can be challenging in the initial stages. This is the reason, why pediatricians and family physicians will direct the patient to the emergency department in case of any mild, unexplained fever, especially in a patient who has recently undergone a shunt insertion or revision. Though this is sometimes prudent, not uncommonly one finds children with obvious throat infection (pharyngitis), ear infection (otitis media), or other infections attending emergency services to rule out shunt infection. However, one should realize that pediatricians are often not experienced enough to diagnose neurosurgical concerns with shunt and hence do not want to miss a shunt infection in its early stages when it can be adequately treated.

The ideal way to diagnose shunt infection is to grow bacteria from the CSF obtained from the shunt. This requires a shunt tap to obtain the CSF and send it to the laboratory for examination. As there have been reports of a negative CSF culture (not growing any bacteria) when the patient is on antibiotics, physicians may hesitate to start a patient on antibiotics before obtaining a culture. However, waiting for the neurosurgeon to arrive and tap the shunt to start antibiotics is sometimes not prudent, considering that shunt infections have never been reported cured with a dose or even a day of antibiotics.

Let us discuss how to interpret the results of the CSF obtained by the shunt tap. The physician usually collects about 5–7 cubic centimeters of CSF and then divides into two or three samples to be sent to the lab. Three groups of tests are usually performed: (a) cell count and differential count (type of cells), (b) glucose and protein level, and (c) Gram's stain and culture. The first two groups of test and the Gram's stain can be done immediately, and the results are sometimes known as quickly as within 30 minutes. We will go through each of them (from the most diagnostic to the least diagnostic) and see how the physicians interpret the results.

Culture: This is the most direct and surest sign of infection. In culture, the microbiologist usually inoculates a few drops of CSF into a medium that supports the bacterial growth (either a culture plate of a broth) and then observes whether bacteria grow in the culture medium. Once the bacteria are identified further, studies are carried out to see to which antibiotics they are sensitive to, which helps the treating physician to choose the ideal antibiotic. As it requires bacteria to grow and then be identified, it takes at least 24 hours to know the preliminary results and 3 or 4 days for the final result. The culture is the most specific test among the panel of tests mentioned. However, cultures can often be negative if the bacteria is too fragile to survive for a short period outside (dies between isolation and processing in the lab) or if appropriate antibiotics are administered before collecting the sample (false-negative result). The latter is often true for blood cultures, but many doctors think it may influence results in CSF cultures also. However, contamination of the sample while collecting or transporting to the lab may result in organisms that are isolated in culture but were not present in the initial sample while collection (false positive result).

Gram's stain

A microbiological laboratory technique. The technique is used as a tool to differentiate between gram-positive and gram-negative bacteria, as a first step to determine the identity of a particular bacterial sample. The word Gram refers to Hans Christian Gram, the inventor of Gram's staining.

Gram's stain: The next most direct evidence is the Gram's stain. Gram's staining is a method of differentiating bacterial species into two large groups (gram positive and gram negative) based on the chemical and physical properties of their cell wall structures. The method is named after its inventor, Danish scientist Hans Gram (1853–1938). This technique was developed in 1884 to differentiate between two types of bacteria-causing pneumonia. The fluid is stained with Gram's stain (crystal violet) and the bacteria are usually differentiated into two groups: gram positive and gram negative. The gram-positive bacteria appear purple (the color of the stain) and the gram-negative cells are pink or red (the color of the counterstain; these bacteria do not retain the crystal violet stain and hence are stained with the counterstain, which is pink).

Most bacteria-causing shunt infection are gram-positive organisms, which are usually rounded organisms called cocci (you may hear about the term gram-positive cocci). However, gram-negative organisms can also cause shunt infection (like gram-negative rods) or may have mixed organisms (mixture of gram-positive and gram-negative bacteria or cocci).

The advantage of Gram's stain is that it provides a quick way to tell, with a certain degree of confidence, whether the shunt infection is present and narrows down to the groups of organisms so that antibiotics can be started on a presumptive basis before the culture results are available. In cases with extremely fragile bacteria or with antibiotic therapy, in which the culture is unable to grow, Gram's stain usually reveals the bacteria, thus aiding in diagnosis. However, Gram's stain is often difficult to interpret and may be interpreted incorrectly with the possibility of both false positives and false negatives. A negative Gram's stain does not rule out a shunt infection unless cultures are corroborated.

White blood cell count and differential count: The CSF is also analyzed for total cell count (including white blood cells and red blood cells) and the differential count. The number of white blood cells in CSF is very low, *less than five cells per high power field*. An increased number of white blood cells (leucocytes) in CSF occurs with infection and is regarded as indirect evidence for infection because an increased cell count can occur in many other conditions, including infection (viral, bacterial, fungal, and parasitic), allergy, leukemia, multiple sclerosis, hemorrhage, and traumatic tap.

To differentiate between these conditions, the differential count on the white blood cells is performed. Usually, a polymorphic response (polymorphs are a type of cells usually present in acute bacterial infection) is seen with bacterial infection, including most shunt infections, while viral infection is usually associated with an increase in lymphocytes (another type of cells). Eosinophils are associated with allergy, while red blood cells are associated with hemorrhage or trauma.

CSF glucose: Normally, CSF contains glucose, which is also reduced in infection. Usually, there is a correlation between blood glucose and CSF glucose, and, in uncertain cases, a disproportionately lower CSF glucose points toward an infection.

CSF glucose

The glucose concentration in the cerebrospinal fluid. It is considerably reduced in bacterial meningitis and helps in corroborating the diagnosis.

However, levels of glucose also can be reduced postoperatively with the presence of blood in the CSF and hence would require correlation with the clinical picture.

CSF protein

The protein concentration in the cerebrospinal fluid.

CSF protein: The protein content in CSF has no direct correlation with acute shunt infection, whereas it may be elevated in a variety of conditions such as the presence of prior bleeding or chronic infections.

Treatment of shunt infection: The aim of treatment is to minimize morbidity and mortality, and to control infection while maintaining CSF drainage.

Shunt infections may require removing the shunt tube and placing in an external drain (to drain the CSF while the infection is being treated with antibiotics and replacing the shunt after complete eradication of infection). Various alterations may be done to the previous regimen, depending on the clinical condition and the location of infection. For example, in a patient with only lower-end wound infection, and no demonstration of bacteria in the ventricular CSF, the shunt can be exteriorized farther up (away from the infected site) and replaced with another shunt once the infection is treated. Sometimes the neurosurgeon would like to insert the shunt on the opposite side, if it is feasible, rather than replace the new shunt on the same side. Intraventricular antibiotics can be administered through the ventriculostomy catheter, thus accelerating the eradication of infection. CSF samples are sent every alternate day, and three consecutive negative culture reports indicate the appropriate time for replacing the shunt. In the presence of a foreign body such as a retained ventricular or peritoneal catheter, an attempt is made to remove it at the time of externalization of the shunt. Antibiotics are continued for several days after insertion of the fresh device.

Occasionally, intravenous antibiotics alone may adequately treat the nonstaphylococcal infections, as these bacteria are not known to colonize the shunt tube. However, because of the low success rate and ultimate requirement for removing the shunt system in 50% of cases, most favor removing the shunt hardware during treatment.

Prevention of shunt infection: Of the various measures advised, systemic prophylactic antibiotics have received the greatest attention. Several studies have concluded that prophylactic systemic antibiotic therapy is indicated for shunt surgery. The antibiotic is administered before the start of the surgery and continued for one day in the postoperative period. Studies have not shown beneficial effect of antibiotics after one day of surgery unless there is higher predisposition for infection (placement of a new shunt after a previous shunt infection, immune deficiencies, or other similar conditions).

Antibiotic impregnated shunt catheters: In the past few years, antibiotic impregnated shunt catheters have been developed. Only one variety is available for clinical use (Bactiseal, Codman). This catheter has two antibiotics: rifampicin and clindamycin, which are effective against gram-positive bacteria (the most common organisms to cause shunt infection) impregnated on the catheter and some of the valves. Preliminary studies have confirmed a significant reduction in shunt infection due to gram-positive organisms in patients with these catheters. However, occasional infections from gram-negative organisms and even from gram-positive organisms have been described with the Bactiseal catheter.

44. Why do shunts overdrain? What is slit ventricle syndrome, and how does it occur?

The most common cause of shunt overdrainage is placement of a low pressure shunt system or siphoning. The two most common effects of overdrainage are (1) occurrence of subdural fluid collection and (2) slit ventricle syndrome.

Because of excessive drainage of the CSF in patients with gross hydrocephalus, the cortical mantle collapses and

Subdural collections

Cerebrospinal fluid or fluid collections in the subdural space (underneath the dura and above the arachnoid). Subdural collections are more prominent in elderly people as the brain shrinks.

Slit ventricle syndrome

A condition associated with slitlike ventricles with symptoms of overdrainage and low-pressure headache. The collapsed ventricles frequently block the proximal catheter leading to shunt obstruction. This is a developmental birth defect, resulting in unused skin, muscles, bone, and spinal cord.

subdural collections develop. These collections often are asymptomatic and do not need any treatment. However, often bleeding occurs into the fluid collections, which requires evacuation. Persistent collections may require replacement of the shunt with a higher-pressure system and an antisiphon device and drainage of the subdural collection. In patients with a programmable shunt, the shunt pressure setting can be raised to obliterate the subdural collection.

In patients without a programmable shunt, inserting a programmable valve with an antisiphon device along with insertion of external subdural drain during the same surgery may be preferable. The programmable valve pressure can be adjusted in the postoperative period to dilate the ventricles, while drainage of subdural fluid is facilitated by the drains that are usually kept in for a few days. The expanded ventricular system ultimately pushes the cortical mantle to the calvarium, thus obliterating the subdural space and the subdural hematoma. After a few weeks, the pressure in the programmable valve can be reduced gradually to effectively manage the hydrocephalus while preventing a redevelopment of the subdural collection.

In **slit ventricle syndrome,** the shunt usually overdrains, causing the ventricles to be small and slitlike. This can be symptomatic presenting in two different ways. Because of overdrainage, the intracranial pressure can be abnormally low, causing symptoms such as headache, nausea, and vomiting, which an erect posture can exacerbate because of the siphon effect. Inserting an antisiphon device or changing to a higher valve pressure may be useful in such conditions.

In the other form of slit ventricle syndrome due to overdrainage, the brain fills the intracranial space and becomes stiff (reduced "compliance"). Thus, it becomes somewhat nonpliable and loses the ability to expand or compress easily. As a result, its ability to compensate for the transient change in intracranial volume is impaired, resulting in relatively large changes in the intracranial pressure. The small ventricles cause intermittent ventricular catheter obstruction as a result of blockage of holes in the catheter by the ependyma and brain matter. These cases usually present with relatively high intracranial pressure with minimal enlargement of the ventricles.

Although small ventricles are often seen, the typical syndrome manifests in only a few patients. In a review of 370 patients, 64% had evidence of slit ventricles in imaging. Only 6.5% had symptoms warranting surgical management (Walker et al., 1993).

Slit ventricle syndrome is one of the most difficult symptoms to treat and is often a nightmare for the pediatric neurosurgeon. Most neurosurgeons will try to avoid a slit ventricle syndrome in susceptible cases by inserting a relatively higher-pressure shunt system initially, which keeps the ventricles relatively open. However, in established patients, various treatment modalities are currently advocated to manage this condition. Conservative treatment includes furosemide, acetazolamide (Diamox), steroids, and antimigranous therapy. In unsuccessful cases, intracranial pressure monitoring and adjusting the shunt valve system to match the intracranial pressure may be preferred. Third ventriculostomy with removal of the shunt has been suggested as an alternative.

45. What are the specific distal end complications of the various types of shunts?

Ventriculoperitoneal Shunt

Ascites: Accumulation of free fluid in the peritoneal cavity is known as ascites. Normally, the peritoneal cavity absorbs the fluid and then returns it to the venous circulation. In ascites, drained CSF is absorbed at a lower rate from the peritoneal cavity, resulting in excess fluid accumulating in the abdominal cavity. The reduced absorption may occur from various causes. A reduced absorbing surface in premature infants often causes

Ascites

This denotes accumulation of free fluid in the peritoneal cavity.

ascites to manifest with abdominal distension after a ventriculoperitoneal shunt insertion. A high protein content of CSF, peritoneal scarring from previous infections, or elevated venous pressure also can result in ascites. Sometimes, it can occur from peritoneal dissemination of malignant brain tumor cells through the shunt tube. Although they are usually sterile, ascites can be infected in as high as 15% of cases. Fluid can become secondarily infected with bloodborne pathogens or by bacteria inoculated at surgery.

Normally, the patient presents with an abdominal distension and bloatedness. Not uncommonly, ascites can present as shunt malfunction due to backpressure and reduction in CSF drainage from the intracranial compartment. Infected ascites are associated with signs of systemic and local infection.

As the entire peritoneum is incompetent in absorbing fluid in ascites, the treatment often is to place the shunt in another cavity such as the atrium. In infected ascites, the shunt is externalized and is placed in an alternate site (atrium, pleura) after the infection has cleared. In premature infants with a reduced absorptive surface, the peritoneum often functions satisfactorily after a year or two.

Pseudoperitoneal cyst

Localized fluid collection in the abdominal (peritoneal) cavity most commonly occurring because of poor absorption of the cerebrospinal fluid drained from a shunt tube.

Pseudoperitoneal cyst: Here, there is a loculated pocket of CSF in the peritoneal cavity, which is usually walled off by bowel and omental tissue. This happens because the CSF is not freely absorbed from the peritoneal cavity and results in a cystic fluid collection that may present as a mass in the abdomen. Mostly, this is associated with a low-grade infection of either the shunt tube or the abdomen, or a previous infection or surgery of the abdominal cavity, resulting in scarring and reduced absorption. Usually, this is easy to diagnose, as the shunt tube is seen lying inside a fluid-filled cavity in the abdomen. The occurrence of a pseudoperitoneal cyst often presents with shunt malfunction and with abdominal distension. Surgery involves exteriorizing the shunt tube, treating the infection if present, and then either reinserting the shunt in another compartment (i.e., converting it into a ventriculoatrial shunt) or in another place in the abdominal cavity. Surprisingly, the second approach works in most patients.

Ascites is differentiated from a pseudoperitoneal cyst by the free movement of fluid in the peritoneal space, whereas it is limited by any membranes (loculated) in the latter. The distinction is significant for few reasons. Pseudoperitoneal cyst is associated with a higher infection rate than ascites. In addition, in ascites, the shunt needs to be removed from the peritoneal cavity, as the entire peritoneal cavity has not been able to absorb fluid, while in the pseudoperitoneal cyst, removing the shunt and replacing it in another region of the peritoneal cavity may suffice.

Ventriculoatrial shunts: In ventriculoatrial shunts, the shunt tube is inserted into the right side of the heart through one of the right neck veins. These shunts are difficult to place and often difficult to revise. However, these shunts are sometimes the only option available in patients with impaired peritoneal absorptive capacity, such as previous peritonitis or premature infants with neonatal enterocolitis. The most significant complication is cardiac failure in young children with gross hydrocephalus, whose cardiac function cannot cope with the extra amount of CSF. Other specific complications include arrhythmia change in the heart rate mostly from a longer tube irritating the heart muscles, pulmonary hypertension, and relatively higher rate and quicker spread of infection into the bloodstream if the shunt becomes infected. In addition, in children, these shunts need to be lengthened more often than peritoneal shunts to accommodate growth.

Ventriculopleural shunts: These shunts use the pleural cavity (the space between the lining membranes of the lungs) as the absorptive surface for spinal fluid. Considering that the pleural space is lesser in surface area in young children and in infants, there is a higher incidence of developing pleural effusion (fluid accumulating in the pleural cavity) in these patients than in adults and older children. Hence, these shunts are often not considered in infants and young children or in patients with compromised pulmonary function, such as kyphoscoliosis, which is often present in patients with myelomeningocele. Other complications include occasional sharp pain on the chest wall, often due to the shunt tube irritating the pleural membrane.

46. A few days after a shunt was inserted in my 6-month-old baby, a fluid pocket appeared under the shunt insertion site in his head. Why did that happen?

CSF leak and peritubal CSF collection is a significant issue in patients with gross hydrocephalus and thin cortical mantle (thickness of the brain tissue) as seen in infants with gross hydrocephalus and in adults with chronic hydrocephalus and large ventricles. After surgery, CSF leaks and collects around the shunt tube, because CSF, like the flow of water, finds it easier to seep around the tube into the subcutaneous plane than to take the pathway of higher resistance—the shunt tube. The thin cortical mantle encourages CSF to seep out of the ventricle, as there is less brain tissue plugging around the tube. This sometime indicates that the resistance in the shunt system is higher than the CSF flow desires and may indicate a subtle shunt malfunction.

With a persistent collection, most often, neurosurgeons will change the shunt system to a relatively lower-pressure system and remove any antisiphon devices they have inserted. Some may apply a mild pressure dressing to avoid fluid collecting in the subgaleal space. Experienced neurosurgeons avoid this problem postoperatively by making a tiny punctate dural opening and avoid creating a very large subgaleal pocket while inserting the shunt valve.

47. What are lumboperitoneal shunts?

In **lumboperitoneal shunts**, the proximal end of the shunt is inserted into the lumbar spinal space, and the distal end is introduced into the peritoneal cavity. Thus, it differs from the conventional ventriculoperitoneal shunt, as it drains the spinal compartment and not the ventricular compartment. The shunt is commonly inserted into the lumbar spinal compartment by a large bore spinal tap needle, is tunneled in the subcutaneous tissue, and is then inserted into the abdominal cavity. On occasion, the surgeon may prefer to perform a laminectomy (removal of the posterior part of the spine) and insert the shunt into the spinal compartment. The surgery is commonly performed in a lateral position. Lumboperitoneal shunts have been performed in communicating hydrocephalus where there is a free communication between intracranial and intraspinal CSF compartments. There have been reports of progressive cerebellar tonsillar herniation with these shunts during follow-up.

Lumboperitoneal shunt

A shunt diverting cerebrospinal fluid from the lumbar region to the abdominal cavity. Usually used as an alternative to ventriculoperitoneal shunt.

Shunt Surgery

PART ELEVEN

Alternatives to Shunting

What are the alternative options to shunt placement?

Can you tell me more about endoscopic third ventriculostomy?

How do aqueductoplasty and aqueductal stenting differ from endoscopic third ventriculostomy?

48. What are the alternative options to shunt placement?

For several decades, shunt placement was the only reasonable surgery to treat hydrocephalus. However, in the past few decades, a few alternative techniques have been used to treat hydrocephalus. We will discuss when each can be used. However, we should always remember that the shunt remains the principal mode of treating hydrocephalus and serves as a backup surgery if any of these procedures fail.

The following options are available as an alternative to shunt:

- Endoscopic third ventriculostomy
- Endoscopic aqueductoplasty
- Endoscopic aqueductal stenting
- Endoscopic septostomy

Before we proceed further we should consider the following:

a. All these alternative procedures are currently only effective in certain type of obstructive hydrocephalus. Recall our discussion about obstructive and communicating hydrocephalus in previous chapters. To recapitulate, in obstructive hydrocephalus, the ventricular CSF does not freely communicate with the subarachnoid CSF. This indicates that an obstruction can be at the level of foramen of Monro, third ventricle, the aqueduct, or at the fourth ventricle or its outlet.

b. These procedures have *two types of failure*: (1) technical failure (the inability to perform the procedure) and (2) procedural failure (the procedure fails to perform its intended job, though it was successfully performed). *Technical failure* is apparent by the completion of the surgery; that is, the surgeon knows whether he could successfully create the communication. The *procedural failure* however, takes longer to know whether a failure has occurred. It may be as early as few days to as late as several years. However, most procedural failures are apparent within six weeks to 3 months, and once the follow-up is well beyond this period, most neurosurgeons would consider it to be successful though late failures may be apparent later.

Emily and Michael's comment:

Our daughter, Christine, was not born with hydrocephalus. Around 10 years of age, she started to complain of mild headaches often toward the end of the school periods. Also the teacher mentioned that she was falling in her grades and was not concentrating. We were worried. Our pediatrician referred us to the pediatric neurologist, who obtained a MRI scan and to our surprise she had huge ventricles. There was obstruction to the CSF flow inside the brain. Our neurosurgeon diagnosed it as aqueductal stenosis and mentioned to us about this procedure "endoscopic third ventriculostomy." He said that it is a very simple procedure which can effectively manage hydrocephalus and if it works well the shunt would not be required. We were initially apprehensive about it but agreed subsequently. The surgery was done and thank God it worked well. Now Christine is 5 years from surgery. She is shunt free and is in 10th grade. Her dream is to become a pediatric neurosurgeon!

49. Can you tell me more about endoscopic third ventriculostomy?

Endoscopic third ventriculostomy was initially practiced in the 1930s but was given up, as the instrumentation was inadequate for this procedure. However, in the late 1980s with the availability of improved instrumentation, better endoscopes with a light source and camera meant a resurgence in endoscopic techniques. Further, the availability of MRI made it possible to visualize preoperatively the obstructive element and thus plan this eloquent CSF diversion procedure.

Anatomical background: It is important to understand the anatomical background and the concept behind this procedure. Normally, CSF flows from the lateral ventricle through the foramen of Monro, through the third ventricle, through the aqueduct to the fourth ventricle, and then exits out via the foramen of Magendie and Luschka to the subarachnoid spaces (Figure 4, p. 12). The endoscopic third ventriculostomy (ETV) is performed by making a fenestration in the floor of the third ventricle, thus diverting fluid from the third ventricle to the basal subarachnoid spaces. Thus, the CSF bypasses before the obstruction (aqueduct, posterior portion of the third ventricle, fourth ventricle) and enters the subarachnoid spaces. Considering this, it will be only effective in conditions in which the obstruction exists between these two points, that is, beyond (distal to) the third ventricle and before (proximal to) the basal subarachnoid spaces. In other words, this will be effective in obstructions at

- Posterior third ventricle (for example, hydrocephalus associated with pineal tumors)
- Aqueduct (most common pathology: aqueductal stenosis)
- Obstruction of the fourth ventricle (tumors in cerebellum or the fourth ventricle)
- Obstruction to the outlet foramina of the fourth ventricle (Dandy-Walker malformation, acquired fourth ventricular outlet obstruction)
- Obstruction at the region of basal cisterns around the cisterna magna (Chiari malformation)

The concept of ETV can be well understood if one takes the example of diversion and flow of traffic around a blocked freeway: We usually take the exit before the blocked segment, travel on the feeder road, and join the freeway after the blocked segment. CSF flowing through the ETV does exactly the same; in a third ventriculostomy, we essentially open the pathway by a fenestration before the blocked segment.

The procedure: Endoscopic third ventriculostomy is performed as an inpatient procedure. The right frontal region is commonly chosen for the entrance into the ventricle and a burr hole is placed. The dural is then opened and the edges are coagulated to prevent any bleeding. The ventricles are then tapped with the help of a brain cannula or a peel-away sheath. The endoscope is introduced into the ventricular cavity, and the anatomical landmarks are identified. The endoscope is introduced into the third ventricle, and the floor is inspected (**Figure 27** and **Figure 28**). The site for the fenestration is chosen in front of the basilar artery (a large artery that supplies blood to the brain) and behind a bony prominence known as the clivus. Usually, the fenestration is performed in the midline although it may swivel to either side (mostly to the left side as the approach is from the right). Fenestration is usually made with blunt perforation, although reportedly a laser has been used. I prefer to use blunt perforation, as it is relatively safer than a laser. A misdirected laser beam can burn a hole in the artery just behind it, causing life-threatening bleeding. The perforation is subsequently dilated using a small balloon catheter (Fogarty catheter) or by passage of the endoscope (**Figure 29**). There can be a mild drop in heart rate during dilatation due to the stimulation of the hypothalamic nuclei (part of the brain responsible for maintaining the heart rate), which reverses itself. The basal cisterns are visualized to see whether fenestration is complete and whether any additional membranes need to be fenestrated. Once the procedure is performed, the endoscope is withdrawn from the ventricular cavity. Most neurosurgeons use lactated Ringer's solution (a type of fluid preparation commonly used as IV fluids) at body temperature to irrigate the ventricles and to wash away any minor bleeding during the procedure. The dural opening is covered with gel foam (a substance used in neurosurgery prevent bleeding) and then the scalp over it is closed. Some surgeons place a titanium cover at the site of the burr hole for cosmetic reasons. The complete procedure takes about 45 minutes with additional time for anesthesia.

Endoscopic third ventriculostomy is performed as an inpatient procedure.

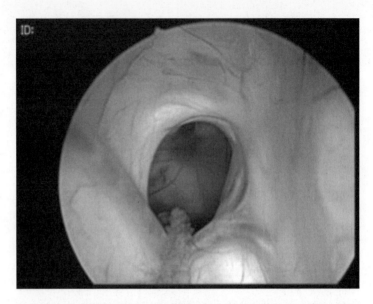

Figure 27. Endoscopic View of the Foramen of Monro and a Glimpse of the Third Ventricle through the Foramen.

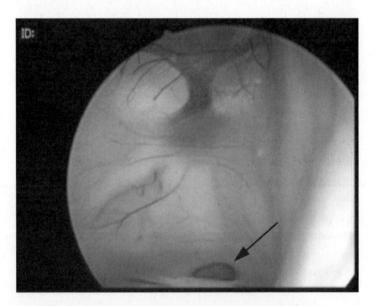

Figure 28. Endoscopic View of the Floor of the Third Ventricle. Note the obstructed aqueduct seen at the six o'clock position. (Arrow)

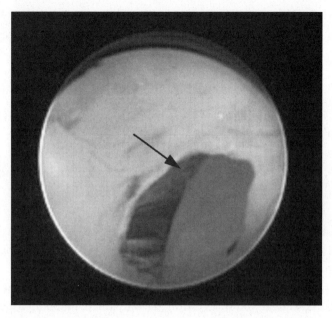

Figure 29. Endoscopic View of the Fenestration During the Third Ventriculostomy. The basilar artery is seen through the fenestration. (Arrow)

Success and failures: A perplexing finding that baffles neurosurgeons is the extreme variation in success rates of endoscopic third ventriculostomy. Why the same surgery works for some and but not others is still unclear. However, by analyzing all procedures performed in the past two decades, we have broad agreement on some areas.

1. **Age:** Age is a significant factor, with success rates varying from as low as 30% in neonates to as high as 90% in adults and children older than 2 years. Age is the single variable all studies agree on.

2. **Cause of hydrocephalus:** The cause of hydrocephalus is another important factor. Success rates are higher in patients without any prior history of infection than in those with infection. Thus, the success rate is low in patients with active infection, whereas it is expected to be high in patients with tumor-related

Alternatives to Shunting

hydrocephalus. Patients with healed infection have intermediate success rates, varying with the nature of the infection. Success rates are also lower in patients who have hydrocephalus with a previous history of hemorrhage.

3.   **Previous shunt surgery:** Endoscopic third ventriculostomy has been successful in patients who have been shunted for hydrocephalus and present with shunt failure. The success rates vary between 40% and 60%.

Early failure and late failure: Early failures occur because diverted spinal fluid is not adequately absorbed by the final absorbing process, although fenestration remains open in most cases. Early failures are most often treated by ventriculoperitoneal shunt insertion, accompanied by endoscopic inspection to confirm patency of the fenestration. However, nonfunctioning of a previously functioning third ventriculostomy several months or years later has been witnessed. Most failures are due to reclosing and rescarring of the fenestration. Fortunately, these reclosures are uncommon, though not infrequent, with the incidence varying between 8% and 15%. An inability to diagnose reclosures can be devastating; a repeat third ventriculostomy can successfully treat reclosures.

Complications of third ventriculostomy: Like any other procedure, endoscopic third ventriculostomy has its share of complications, including bleeding during the procedure, infection, brain injury, and failure of the procedure. Unique complications for this are enumerated in the subsequent paragraphs.

1.   **Bleeding from the basilar artery or its branches:** The procedure is performed in the third ventricular floor in front of the basilar artery. The chances of injuring the artery are low if the neurosurgeon visualizes the artery during surgery. However, several reports have described injury of the artery, resulting in mortality. One late complication of patients who survive is

development of a pseudoaneurysm formation in the basilar artery (the injury to the wall causes development of abnormal dilatation). In this regard, the neurosurgeon will usually follow up with an angiogram or magnetic resonance angiogram to see whether an aneurysm has developed.

2. **CSF leak:** Leakage of spinal fluid through the operative site is common after an endoscopic third ventriculostomy. This is more frequent in infants and young children with thin cerebral mantle (thickness of the brain) and essentially presents within the first few days of surgery. Most of the time, a profuse leak is associated with an early failure, as CSF finds it easier to leak into the subcutaneous tissue and through the sutures than to be absorbed in the system. However, an improperly closed wound has a higher predilection of leaking and may not suggest failure. The leak is sometimes managed by resuturing the wound, which increases resistance to the CSF flow into the wound and encourages the CSF to flow through the normal absorptive system.

3. **Hypothalamic injury and endocrine disturbances:** Hypothalamic and endocrine disturbances often have been reported from damage to the hypothalamic nuclei. Most often it results if fenestration is slightly eccentric than central. However, this is uncommon and can be managed with hormone supplementation.

4. **Subdural collection:** Subdural collections are much less commonly associated with endoscopic CSF diversion procedures such as third ventriculostomy than with ventriculoperitoneal shunt because the CSF flows across a normal physiologic pressure head. Fortunately, subdural collections are minimal and managed with observation.

5. **Double vision, ptosis:** Injury to the cranial nerves during the procedure can result in double vision and sometimes drooping eyelid. These are uncommon but have been reported.

50. How do aqueductoplasty and aqueductal stenting differ from endoscopic third ventriculostomy?

In suitable cases, endoscopic aqueductoplasty and aqueductal stenting are exciting alternatives to endoscopic third ventriculostomy. **Aqueductoplasty** basically means opening up the obstructed aqueduct. Because it is done under endoscopic guidance, it is called an endoscopic aqueductoplasty. However, in **aqueductal stenting**, the aqueduct is opened up (aqueductoplasty) and a permanent thin tube (stent) is placed across the aqueduct to prevent the aqueductoplasty from closing.

Anatomical background: Two procedures are only suitable in a select group of patients. To understand the indications for these procedures, we have to revisit the "circuit diagram" of the CSF pathway. These procedures are only suitable in obstructive hydrocephalus and not in communicating hydrocephalus. Further, not all types of obstructive hydrocephalus are suitable for the procedure. As these procedures involve opening of the aqueduct, of all types of obstructive hydrocephalus, only patients with an obstructed aqueduct would be suitable. Further, with an obstructed aqueduct, not all patients will be suitable. If we realize the anatomy of aqueduct, it is a relatively long and narrow channel a few millimeters in diameter. With the advent of MRI, we now know that there are several types of aqueductal stenosis, depending on the extent and degree of the obstruction. Of the several types of aqueductal stenosis, most endoscopic neurosurgeons consider only a subgroup of aqueductal stenosis in which this procedure can be safely performed. Patients with **aqueductal web** (a thin membrane blocking the aqueduct) and those with a **short segment stenosis** (less than 5 millimeter length of a segment stenosed) are considered to

Aqueductoplasty

A surgical procedure, where usually by an endoscopic route, the blocked segment of the aqueduct is dilated by using a small inflatable balloon.

Aqueductal stenting

A surgical procedure, where usually by an endoscopic route, a thin tube (stent) is placed in the aqueduct across the stenosed segment to maintain the cerebrospinal fluid flow from the third to the fourth ventricle.

Aqueductal web

A form of aqueductal stenosis in which a thin web of tissue blocks the cerebrospinal fluid flow across the aqueduct.

Short segment aqueductal stenosis

A type of aqueductal stenosis in which the aqueduct is obstructed only for a short segment of its length.

be ideal candidates (**Figure 30**). Patients with long segment stenosis (more than 5 millimeter stenosed segment) are usually not considered for the procedure, as brain stem injury (the area of the brain anterior and posterior to the aqueduct) is possible with the present technology (**Figure 31**).

The procedure: The procedure is essentially similar to the endoscopic third ventriculostomy with the exception that the burr hole is placed more anteriorly than the conventional burr hole for the endoscopic third ventriculostomy. The endoscope is advanced into the lateral, into the third, and then into the aqueductal inlet. The aqueduct is inspected, and, considering the preoperative MRI scan, a decision is made about whether the aqueduct can be fenestrated safely (**Figure 32**). If it can be, a fenestration is made using a 3 French Fogarty catheter and the balloon is subsequently inflated.

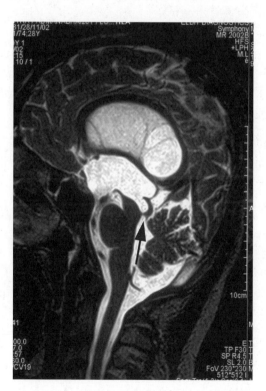

Figure 30. Preoperative MRI Demonstrating an Aqueductal Web. (Arrow)

Most of the time, the preoperative imaging will have either demonstrated a short segment stenosis of a web blocking the aqueduct. Both of these are often associated with a pinhole opening carefully cannulated with the Fogarty catheter. Extreme care is taken during the procedure not to injure the lips of the aqueduct. Once an adequate fenestration is made, the Fogarty catheter is withdrawn and the adequacy of fenestration is confirmed. Most will advance the endoscope to have a glimpse of the fourth ventricle cavity, while some others will insert a thinner flexible endoscope (equivalent to a thin ball pen refill diameter) to enter into the aqueduct and visualize the fourth ventricle cavity.

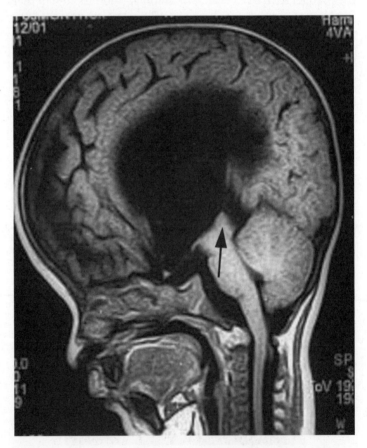

Figure 31. MRI of a Long Segment Aqueductal Stenosis. (Arrow)

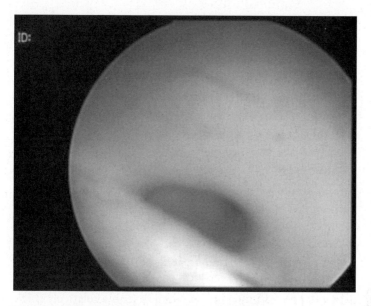

Figure 32. Endoscopic View of a Stenosed Aqueduct.

Once the fenestration is made and is successful, if an aqueductal stent is planned, a thin catheter equivalent to the diameter of the ventricular catheter is passed either through or along the endoscope and placed in the aqueduct with the distal holes in the fourth ventricle. If this is a free stent (without any attachment to any structures), then the proximal end stays in the third ventricle, resting on the aqueductal lip. However, with a fixed stent, the other end is usually attached to a subcutaneous Ommaya reservoir (a small bubble) that secures it, preventing it from migrating from its ideal position. In addition, it serves as a port to drain the CSF and measures the intracranial pressure if required in future.

Complications: Apart from the usual complications common with other intracranial procedures (bleeding, infection, seizures, brain injury), there are some specific complications associated with aqueductal injury, including double vision, drooping of eyelid, squinting, and occasionally unresponsiveness. Reclosure is a significant long-term complication associated with aqueductoplasty, and stents can either migrate or close.

Efficacy of aqueductoplasty and aqueductal stenting: The first question that comes to mind is whether both procedures have a better outcome than endoscopic third ventriculostomy. Unfortunately, not enough data exist in the current literature to indicate whether these procedures are better than endoscopic third ventriculostomy. Some preliminary data indicate that these are probably as efficacious as endoscopic third ventriculostomy. However, these procedures are only considered in a highly selective group of patients who are carefully chosen before surgery, and we have no large clinical trials or randomized control trials for this.

However, in certain patients it can be performed when third ventriculostomy is contraindicated. For example, with a very narrow prepontine space (the basilar artery is quite close and is in a danger of injury) or in patients with a relatively thick nontransparent floor where endoscopic third ventriculostomy cannot be considered, aqueductoplasty or aqueductal stenting may be an option.

PART TWELVE

Follow–Up of Patients with Shunts

Does this shunt last for a lifetime or does it need to be changed?

Can I follow up with my family doctor or pediatrician instead of seeing my neurosurgeon? Can something happen in the period before my next follow-up?

Are shunt malfunctions considered emergencies?

More...

It is obvious that you would have several questions about an indwelling shunt. In this chapter, we shall try to answer some commonly asked questions concerning the follow-up of the shunted patient.

51. Is the shunt requirement permanent or, in other words, "once a shunt, always a shunt?"

Most often, this statement holds true. However, with availability of newer techniques for treating hydrocephalus, shunt dependency can be reversed in some cases. Let's describe some circumstances in which we can remove the shunt or make the person shunt independent.

In some circumstances, after placement of the shunt, there is a possibility that the initial pathology that caused the hydrocephalus either resolves or is adequately treated. A prime example is hydrocephalus associated with tumor in which the tumor is the initial pathology that causes obstruction of the CSF pathway, resulting in hydrocephalus. In such cases after complete removal of the tumor, the obstruction is reversed and the shunt may no longer be required and may be removed. However, in most circumstances, the pathways do not reopen completely, resulting in drainage of some CSF through the shunt. This makes the brain stay "dependent on the shunt" as CSF flows comparatively easily through the shunt than through the normal pathway. During a follow-up evaluation a year later, it is difficult for the surgeon to estimate the amount of CSF flowing through the shunt and through the normal pathways. In an asymptomatic patient with small ventricles and an intact shunt, it is justified to assume drainage of CSF by the shunt, indicating that the shunt is required. Under these circumstances, the neurosurgeon would opine that the shunt is required. However, if the shunt is disconnected or has migrated and the patient is asymptomatic with evidence of small ventricles in the CT scan, it is inferred that the shunt may not be required and it may be removed. However, most neurosurgeons watch carefully for symptoms to develop and decide about the requirement at a subsequent follow-up. 3 months later, assuming that the patient remains asymptomatic, the neurosurgeon may remove the shunt. Some neurosurgeons may leave it in place, knowing that it is not functioning or not required, simply because the retained shunt tube does not cause any concerns and its removal would require another operation. Apart from tumor-related hydrocephalus, a similar situation may be seen in hydrocephalus associated with infections and subarachnoid hemorrhage. Similarly, a subduroperitoneal shunt may be removed in children with benign external hydrocephalus once the condition resolves.

Now, let us discuss another scenario. The patient with obstructive hydrocephalus has had a shunt placed several years before. Because of newer technologies and available alternatives to shunting, we can possibly make this patient shunt independent by performing an endoscopic third ventriculostomy and removing the shunt postoperatively. However, the shunt is usually removed after confirming that the endoscopic procedure is functioning adequately and the patient no longer requires the shunt (weaning of the shunt).

Considering the previous discussion, we can assume that almost 90–95% of shunt requirements are permanent. In a recent French study, only 4.2% of 1,564 children were weaned from shunts. However, it is imperative that we identify the 5–10% of patients in whom the shunt is not required and can be removed, as it significantly reduces follow-up requirement with a neurosurgeon and reduces emergency room visits. Therefore, most neurosurgeons have a relatively high threshold for inserting shunts and would consider temporary methods of CSF diversion (like external ventricular drainage) for conditions in which the CSF diversion requirement may not be permanent.

52. Does this shunt last for a lifetime, or does it need to be changed?

The simple answer is no.

No mechanical device can function for a lifetime, and, unfortunately, shunts fall into this group.

So how long does a shunt last? This is a difficult question. Shunt tubes are made of high-quality silicon and last for several years, sometimes as long as 10–15 years. However, most shunt tubes are replaced before this period because of either malfunction or other conditions. About 82% of shunts fail within 12 years of insertion; the malfunction rate for the first year is approximately 30%.

Over the years, shunts disintegrate because of degradation of silicone to silica by the body's immune system. During the growth years (when the child usually gains height), degraded catheters adhere to subcutaneous tissue, thus failing to unreel from the peritoneal cavity. Continuous stretching of the brittle catheters causes them to rupture and disconnect, causing the shunt to migrate. If a neurosurgeon is revising the shunt for other reasons, the surgeon will also change to a new tube if the tube is at least a year old, although some may reuse the previously inserted shunt.

53. At what intervals and for how long will follow-up be required? What investigations are to be done at follow-up?

The duration of follow-up monitoring is lifelong because shunt obstructions can occur as late as 20 years after insertion and successful functioning.

The first evaluation ideally should be between 6 weeks and 3 months of the insertion or revision of the shunt. This is essential because it takes 6 to 8 weeks for ventricles to reduce. A CT or MRI scan (usually a CT scan) is performed to assess the baseline status of the ventricles (**Figure 33**). This is considered essential as the baseline ventricular size is used as a reference for comparison in the future when the shunt malfunctions (**Figure 34**). I usually prefer the CT scan to be performed in the same hospital or hospital group where the patient is likely to be evaluated when the shunt malfunctions. Having the baseline CT scan in the same hospital allows the CT scan to be reviewed quickly, thus reducing the lag time when it matters most. Most hospitals have an electronic radiology viewing system (PACS) to permit off-site viewing access to its physicians. This allows your neurosurgeon to view and compare the shunt from his home if required. This is highly beneficial in circumstances where it is required most, that is, in the emergency room. I also stress that families keep a copy of the baseline CT (done at six-week follow-up) with them, which can be useful if the shunt malfunctions while they are traveling. The 6- to 12-week follow-up also assesses improvement of symptoms and indicates which symptoms are less likely to improve after the surgery.

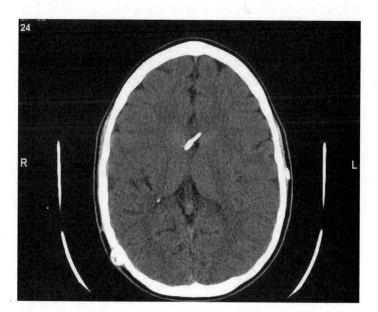

Figure 33. CT Scan of Well Decompressed Ventricle by a Shunt.

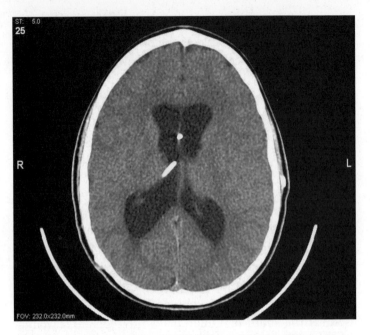

Figure 34. CT Scan of Malfunctioning Shunt with Dilated Ventricles.

Subsequent follow-ups are somewhat controversial. This does not mean that follow-ups are not required, but there is disagreement about intervals of follow-ups. Most neurosurgeons like to reevaluate in 6 to nine 9 time (i.e., one year after the surgery) and then once a year. However, earlier follow-ups are arranged in special circumstances, such as to reprogram the shunt. Some neurosurgeons opt to follow up at 2–3 years because the shunt may malfunction at any time, even a day after the last regular follow-up. A noncontrast CT scan and a shunt series (several overlapping X-rays of the head, neck, chest, and abdomen to see the integrity and continuity of the shunt tube) are done during these follow-ups. These follow-ups are required to detect any asymptomatic shunt malfunctions or any breakage and discontinuation of the shunt tube.

54. Can I follow up with my family doctor or pediatrician instead of seeing my neurosurgeon? Can something happen in the period before my next follow-up?

This is a valid question that has no straight answers. There have been some efforts to redirect follow-up care of patients with hydrocephalus to pediatricians or family practitioners to reduce the burden on neurosurgeons. However, most neurosurgeons would be uncomfortable with the primary care physician or pediatricians evaluating patients for the follow-up. Neurosurgeons and pediatric neurosurgeons look for symptoms and signs that often can be missed in a pediatrician's or a family practitioner's routine evaluation. In addition, follow-up evaluations are required to evaluate outcomes, redefine indications, and optimize treatment as new technologies develop. Annual or biannual contact with the family and the growing child is a great opportunity for the neurosurgeon to maintain a rapport with the family and to answer their questions as newer technologies arrive and alternate treatment options are defined. From the patient's standpoint, it permits patients and families to be reinformed regarding signs and symptoms of shunt malfunction, to get any new information or treatment options since the last surgery, and, most important, to have access to timely medical care when the shunt malfunctions. Thus, it is common for neurosurgeons to evaluate an asymptomatic patient with a functioning shunt who has recently relocated to be familiar with his clinical condition and establish a rapport.

In the intervening period, the shunt may have failed or become infected. Shunt infections are uncommon after 6 months of initial insertion (see Question 56). However, shunt malfunctions can happen anytime, even a day after the shunt is inserted. It is imperative to know the features of shunt malfunction or infection so that you can recognize them early.

55. Are shunt malfunctions considered emergencies?

Yes, shunt malfunctions are invariably treated as emergencies. You may come across chronic shunt malfunction in which the shunt is partially functioning. Hence, once diagnosed the patient is immediately transferred to neurosurgical care and often the neurosurgeon is the best person to decide when to intervene.

56. Can this shunt get infected and, if so, when?

Although theoretically shunt infections can occur at anytime, they are usually seen within the first 6 months of insertion. Most shunt infections occur during shunt insertion surgery. Bacteria, which commonly cause shunt infection, are either *Staphylococcus epidermidis* or *Staphylococcus aureus*. Although the *Staphylococcus epidermidis* infection is acquired during insertion, it usually manifests several weeks or months after insertion because the slowly multiplying bacteria attach to the tube and form a slimy layer covering the tube. Subsequently, it slowly infects the CSF. Infection with *Staphylococcus aureus* is usually quicker and often manifests within a few weeks of the insertion.

Although theoretically shunt infections can occur at anytime, they are usually seen within the first six months of insertion.

However, infection can still occur several years later if the shunt has been recently tapped, or there has been spread and dissemination of bacteria through the bloodstream. The latter can lead to bacteria settling on the shunt tube, causing infection. Some doctors and dentists routinely administer antibiotics before any procedure in which bacteria might be disseminated (see Question 63).

57. Is my shunt guaranteed to function?

As it is impossible to predict how long kitchen plumbing pipes will remain unclogged, no neurosurgeon can guarantee how long the shunt can remain patent. If you have a guarantee from your surgeon, do not look forward to it, as it is invariably a void guarantee.

58. I have a programmable valve in my shunt. What precautions do I have to take?

The flow through the programmable valves is controlled by an external regulator that provides a powerful external magnet to adjust the existing pressure setting. The pressure setting in some of the valves get deranged by MRI scan, which uses a powerful magnet to get the images. The Codman Hakim Programmable Valve System and the Medtronic Strata valves fall into this category. However, the Sophysa programmable valves and the Aesculap programmable valves have a safety locking mechanism that prevents damage with an external magnetic force.

If you have one of these valves whose pressure setting is altered with MRI, it is advisable to speak to your neurosurgeon before the MRI to arrange for a convenient time to reset the valve pressure following the MRI. Under emergency circumstances, inform your doctor who has requested the MRI to arrange for a neurosurgeon to reset your pressure setting. It is desirable that you know the valve pressure setting and record it in an accessible place so that the neurosurgeon can reset it to the previous pressure.

PART THIRTEEN

Follow–Up of Patients with Hydrocephalus Without a Shunt

What are the follow-up requirements for endoscopic third ventriculostomy?

What are the follow-up requirements for aqueductoplasty and aqueductal stenting?

My son has been diagnosed with hydrocephalus. However, the neurosurgeon is watching him closely, as he feels he has compensated hydrocephalus. What are the follow-up requirements?

59. What are the follow-up requirements for endoscopic third ventriculostomy?

In patients with endoscopic third ventriculostomy, I usually prefer an MRI to be done at 6 weeks follow-up with special sequences to look for the CSF flow through the third ventricular floor. This is essential as the third ventriculostomy opening can close by scar tissue formation. Although most of the closure occurs in the initial few weeks to months, several reports have described its late closure. Presence of flow void (evidence of CSF flow) confirms the patency of the opening although it does not indicate whether the third ventriculostomy is functioning (i.e., if the CSF is being absorbed by the arachnoid granulations after passing though the opening) (**Figure 35**). Because of occasional reports of late closure of the third ventriculostomy opening after its initial successful functioning, MRI is preferably performed once a year or so.

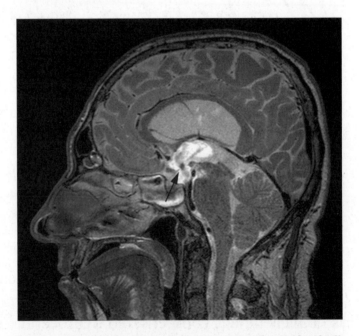

Figure 35. Sagittal MRI of the Brain Demonstrating Flow Void at the Site of Third Ventriculostomy Suggesting a Patent Third Ventriculostomy.

60. What are the follow-up requirements for aqueductoplasty and aqueductal stenting?

The follow-up of nonshunted patients is somewhat different from management of nonshunted patients. As there is no shunt, the follow-up with shunt series is one aspect that differs from the follow-up with shunted patients. Let us discuss each surgical procedure and the follow-up considerations required for each.

1. **Aqueductoplasty:** The single follow-up concern in aqueductoplasty is closure of the aqueductoplasty. The patient usually manifests with symptoms of hydrocephalus as if it was before the surgery. The follow-up imaging required is usually an MRI scan with some specific imaging to look for patency of the aqueductoplasty. Flow of CSF is picked up well by the MRI as it casts "a flow void" and can be quantified by special software. The initial MRI is usually performed in six weeks and then repeated at 6-month intervals and then at yearly intervals. Alternatively, a CT scan with contrast injection can be performed and the flow of the contrast can be confirmed by the CT scan. However, it is an invasive procedure, and the contrast needs to be introduced into the ventricle. A noncontrast CT scan would reflect the degree of hydrocephalus and can indirectly indicate whether the fenestration is open.

2. **Aqueductal stenting:** The follow-up of aqueductal stenting is similar to aqueductoplasty but has some slight differences. The concern with aqueductal stenting is either migration of the stent or blockage of the stent. Usually a radio-opaque catheter is placed, so that its position can be easily identified by a CT scan or even with a plain X-ray of the skull. The stent patency is slightly more difficult to prove with an MRI (**Figure 36**). However, specific flow studies can be conducted to see the flow void through the stent,

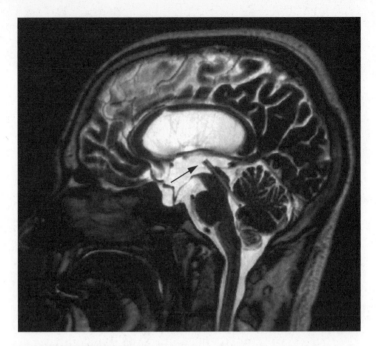

Figure 36. MRI Scan Demonstrating an Aqueductal Stent. (Arrow)

which suggests CSF flowing through it. Alternatively, a CT scan with contrast injected in the ventricles can demonstrate the flow through the stent. However, we should realize that these procedures are in their infancy, and we will know more about them as more procedures are performed.

61. My son has been diagnosed with hydrocephalus. However, the neurosurgeon is watching him closely, as he feels he has compensated hydrocephalus. What are the follow-up requirements?

At times, hydrocephalus is in the mild to moderate range, and a decision is made to closely observe the ventriculomegaly by the treating neurosurgeon. Hence, it is common to find a significant number of patients with ventriculomegaly who are initially managed nonoperatively. These patients need to be followed up closely at least for the initial few months to a year to make sure that symptoms and hydrocephalus do not worsen. The frequency and the duration of follow-up vary in infants and in young children (in whom the fontanel is open) and in older children and adults (in whom the fontanel is closed).

1. **Infants and young children with open fontanel:** The closure of the fontanel and sutures is the single key factor that determines the degree of hydrocephalus. The openings of sutures allow the head to grow in size and compensate for the increased intracranial pressure by slowly enlarging the ventricular size. Head size grows abnormally, though slowly, over the follow-up period. Hence, these patients can be satisfactorily followed up with head circumference measurement. The status of the fontanel can be assessed for the first year or so by clinical evaluation. Head ultrasound through the open fontanel also can be performed at intervals to assess the ventricular size. CT and MRI scans are reserved in cases that require more detailed evaluation or are possible candidates for surgical procedure. Developmental assessment can also be performed once the child is at least 6 months of age. In this age group, the brain is still developing. It is important to pick up subtle signs early. After a follow-up at 4 to 6 weeks, then evaluations are performed at 3-month intervals for at least a year. Subsequent evaluations may be done at 6-month intervals for a year, and if the patient is stable, then yearly follow-ups are sufficient.

2. **Older children with closed fontanel:** The closed fontanel and relatively fused sutures in this age group indicate that the head sizes will unlikely increase with increased pressure. Most children thus develop signs of raised intracranial pressure. However, some

do not show signs of increased pressure and manifest with features of slow deterioration of scholastic performance and progressive stiffness in the lower limbs and gait difficulty. The follow-up evaluation should include a thorough clinical history and neurologic evaluation. Questioning parents regarding the child's overall school performance school as compared with his or her peers is helpful. A CT scan to assess any increase in ventricular size is commonly considered. However, often the CT scan may remain unchanged, thus leading to an erroneous diagnosis of stable ventriculomegaly. A detailed neuropsychologic evaluation by an experienced neuropsychologist is often essential to demonstrate any deterioration of the cognitive and scholastic performance and should be included in the follow up assessments. After an initial 6 months evaluation, an annual follow up with a neuropsychologic evaluation and a noncontrast head CT scan suffices in this group.

In adults, memory, judgment, and other cognitive functions worsen. These are noticed at the workplace where the person fails to keep up with requirements. In addition, there can be subtle gait disturbances as evidenced by a relatively broad-based, short stepping gait accompanied by frequent falls. This may be accompanied by urgency of micturition or incontinence in late stages. Hence, a good clinical history and evaluation accompanied by a neuropsychologic evaluation is essential. The follow-up frequency and duration is similar to the previous group (i.e., initially at 6 months and then yearly).

PART FOURTEEN

Special Circumstances with Indwelling Shunts

How does the presence of the shunt influence surgery for these conditions?

I have a functioning ventriculoperitoneal shunt. Can I undergo peritoneal dialysis?

How do you manage a patient with arrested hydrocephalus?

More...

62. My son has a shunt that is functioning well. Can he participate in contact sports?

Conventionally, it is assumed that children with hydrocephalus and shunts have an increased risk for neurologic injury while participating in contact sports. This is due to several predisposing factors. The reduced brain reserve due to previous insult to the brain makes it less likely to recover from an injury. Children with hydrocephalus often have a thinner skull bone than normal children, thus making them increasingly susceptible to injury while participating in contact sports. In long-standing cases, relatively rigid shunt tubes are more likely to fracture and disconnect. The most significant concern is that these children have larger ventricles than normal populations despite functioning shunts. A relatively larger ventricle and a thinner cortical mantle favor a larger and speedier accumulation of blood in the extracerebral space (e.g., subdural hematoma), as the brain parenchyma can collapse more easily than in patients with a normal parenchyma.

However, an effort should be made to normalize the activities of children with hydrocephalus, as practicable. Participation in organized sports plays an important part in childhood development and contributes to improved physical fitness, self-esteem, and personal discipline in life.

In a previous survey among pediatric neurosurgeons, it was found that sports-related problems in association with ventriculoperitoneal shunts occur, though at an incidence less than 1% (Blount et al., 2004). The most common problems were shunt fractures and shunt dysfunction occurring close to the participation in sports. The other reported problems were occurrence of subdural hematoma in patients with enlarged ventricles. Fracture of the shunt tube also was noted with some reporting hearing a distinct, audible "snap."

Although currently there are no set guidelines for children participating in sports, 89% of surveyed neurosurgeons did not restrict participation in noncontact sports. Approximately one-third of neurosurgeons did not restrict participation in contact sports. Among contact sports, football, boxing, and wrestling were specifically prohibited.

63. I have a functioning shunt. I need to have surgery. What are my additional concerns due to the indwelling shunt?

Often patients with ventriculoperitoneal shunts require other surgical procedures. It is common for the neurosurgeon to be asked about the safety of the procedure before it is contemplated. The circumstances can be broadly divided into the following:

a. Surgeries on patients in which the shunt tube is not exposed

b. Surgeries on patients in which the shunt tube will be or may be exposed

Surgeries on patients in which the shunt tube is not exposed: These procedures should not pose any concern to the shunt's functioning. However, the risk of shunt infection is a potential concern, and the risk is higher if the surgery is performed through a contaminated field such as the oral cavity (e.g., tooth extraction or other dental procedures) and the lower gastrointestinal tract (e.g., colonoscopy, colorectal biopsy) with a predisposition for bacterial dissemination.

Antibiotic prophylaxis for dental procedures: Antibiotic prophylaxis is commonly considered before dental procedures in patients with ventriculoperitoneal and ventriculoatrial shunts. Commonly, a broad-spectrum antibiotic such as *amoxicillin* is administered an hour before the procedure. In patients who are allergic to penicillin, either oral *clindamycin* or intravenous *cefazolin* is administered. The argument for antibiotic prophylaxis before dental procedures is based on the incidence of shunt infection in general and potential devastating consequences. A

Antibiotic prophylaxis

This indicates antibiotics administered for prevention of infection (e.g., during surgery, during hospitalization).

recent review of the literature did not find any adequate data to support this notion (Lockhart et al., 2007). It was also noted that, despite the lack of scientific data, most neurosurgeons recommend that antibiotic prophylaxis may be beneficial for invasive dental procedures. Some others recommend administering antibiotics only for ventriculoatrial shunts and not for ventriculoperitoneal shunts, as the ventriculoatrial shunts are prone to infection.

Surgeries in patients in which the shunt tube will be exposed or may be exposed: This group presents some concerns of the functioning of the shunt in the postoperative period, as the shunt tube is expected to be exposed during the procedure. Exposure of the shunt tube also increases the likelihood of shunt infection either due to dissemination or due to direct contamination during the surgery. Such procedures include abdominal surgeries with an indwelling ventriculoperitoneal shunt and thoracic surgeries with ventriculopleural shunt. Preoperative discussion with a neurosurgeon and the presence of the neurosurgeon in the operating room is considered ideal under such circumstances.

64. How does the presence of the shunt influence surgery for these conditions?

Shunts and appendicitis: Appendicitis is a common condition in pediatric populations, and it is common to find patients with shunts attending the emergency room with appendicitis. In shunted patients, there is a possibility of mistaking the diagnosis: appendicitis being diagnosed as shunt obstruction or vice versa. In addition, the associated vomiting, irritability, fever, and tenderness in the lower-right quadrant may be mistaken for a lower-end shunt infection. These diagnostic errors are common and often delay appropriate treatment.

Uncomplicated appendicitis often can be effectively managed by conventional management protocols. If the shunt tube is seen during the appendectomy, then these often can be managed with replacing the catheter away from the operative site. These children need to be followed up closely to assess for any chronic abdominal infection that may present several weeks after the initial surgery.

Patients with ruptured appendicitis most often need their shunts externalized with intravenous antibiotics. Once the peritoneal infection is settled, another site in the peritoneal cavity can be chosen to insert the shunt. Alternatively, a ventriculoatrial or a ventriculopleural shunt can be considered.

Hernia, hydrocele, and shunts: It is common to see an infant with a shunt-developing hydrocele or hernia a few months after insertion of the shunt. A prior study reported 15% of shunted children developed inguinal hernias, and hydroceles were seen in another 6% of males (Clarnette, 1998). Normally, in utero, there is a patent communication between the abdominal cavity and the scrotum known as the peritoneovaginal canal, which closes in the early neonatal period. Persistence of this canal can cause the CSF to track from the peritoneal cavity into the scrotum, thus causing hydrocele. If the communication is large, bowel loops can migrate into the scrotal sac, resulting in inguinal hernia. In 30% of premature infants and neonates, the passage is patent, thus the infant is at risk for developing hernia or hydrocele. The collection is lax and supple. A tense collection can result due to a slit valve mechanism with one-way CSF flow. The distal end of the shunt tube can migrate into the sac. In most cases, these spontaneously reduce in size and do not need any surgical intervention. However, tense or growing collections need a repositioning of the catheter with correction of the defect.

65. I have a functioning ventriculoperitoneal shunt. Can I undergo peritoneal dialysis?

There are not enough studies in the literature about peritoneal dialysis in patients with ventriculoperitoneal shunts (Warady, 2007). Some authors consider the presence of a ventriculoperitoneal shunt a relative contraindication to peritoneal dialysis because of the potential risk of ascending infection through the shunt and shunt-induced peritoneal damage. Although shunts have one-way valves to prevent reflux of fluid into the ventricles from the peritoneal cavity, there are potential risks of spread of infection from the peritoneal to the ventricular cavity. The second issue in peritoneal dialysis is about the efficacy of the peritoneal membrane secondary to chronic CSF exposure. However, most authors conclude that peritoneal dialysis is not an absolute contraindication in patients with a functioning ventriculoperitoneal shunt; hence, it should not be precluded. It is also not routinely recommended to switch the peritoneal end of the shunt to another compartment such as the pleural cavity and the atrium before initiating peritoneal dialysis.

66. I have had several shunt revisions since childhood. During my last surgery, the neurosurgeon could not take out the peritoneal catheter and left part of the catheter in the subcutaneous tissue. Can it cause problems?

This is a common occurrence, particularly in adults and adolescents who have had shunts since childhood. After several months of insertion, an inflammatory reaction occurs around the shunt tube, which results in formation of a scar tissue track along the tube. Changes in the substance of the catheter (catheters are made of silicone polymer that slowly degrades to silica) make them stiff. This combination leads to breakage of the catheter, which then slowly migrates into the abdominal compartment. The scar tissue track around the catheter acts as a conduit and channels the CSF for some time. However, it ultimately fails, leading to features of shunt malfunction.

Catheters that are barium impregnated are more likely to degenerate than catheters that do not have barium. Barium impregnation is common, as it makes the shunt tube identifiable in

X-rays so that the integrity and continuity can be easily assessed during follow-ups. However, barium is slowly released into the surrounding tissue and incites an inflammatory reaction, resulting in a scar tissue track along the length of the tube.

Managing the retained peritoneal catheters has been somewhat controversial. Most neurosurgeons leave them in the peritoneal cavity, as they do not cause any problems and are well tolerated (**Figure 37**). However, these usually behave as retained foreign bodies and need to be removed if the peritoneal cavity becomes infected. Elective removal has been recommended with laparoscopic techniques but is not widely practiced.

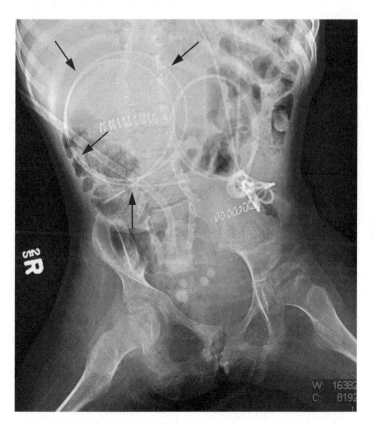

Figure 37. Retained Shunt Tube in the Abdomen. In addition to the shunt tube, which is in continuity, there is another free-floating tube in the abdomen. (Arrows)

67. How do you manage a patient with arrested hydrocephalus?

Although commonly used, arrested hydrocephalus is a controversial terminology in neurosurgical literature. It usually indicates a condition in which the patient has large ventricles in imaging studies, but the CSF production and absorption are well balanced, thus leading to "arrest" of the symptomatology. It is sometimes used in patients who have large ventricles and often a large head but are stable neurologically. However, the subtle balance between the production and absorption often changes, and in such cases, neurologic deterioration often occurs. Any mild change in the CSF dynamics such as a minor head trauma or viral infection can change it to a symptomatic hydrocephalus. For these reasons, many neurosurgeons prefer the term *compensated hydrocephalus* because *arrested* often gives some sort of false security to neurologists, family physicians, or internists.

In a previous study, patients in whom the clinical diagnosis of arrested hydrocephalus was made were found to have decreases in intelligence quotient and had raised intracranial pressure while being monitored. These authors in fact suggested that there may be a very low incidence of true arrested hydrocephalus. In another study, of the 17 patients who underwent CSF diversion procedures, all but one clinically improved during the follow up. Considering these, it is very important that these patients should be monitored closely and a CSF diversion procedure should be considered when in doubt. Neuropsychologic assessments are often useful in assessing subtle worsening in cognitive functions when the neurologic functions are relatively stable.

Recently another term *long-standing overt ventriculomegaly in adult* has been proposed by some. The term long-standing overt ventriculomegaly in adults is self-explanatory, as it indicates an adult with dilated ventricles that has been present over a prolonged period with many having symptoms from infancy or childhood. However, these patients are typically symptomatic with subnormal intelligence quotient, gait difficulty, memory impairment, and urinary symptoms. Some patients may also have tremors. Most patients have noncommunicating hydrocephalus. These patients will need some CSF diversion procedure for their hydrocephalus. Although endoscopic third ventriculostomy has been recommended, a recent report mentions that these patients often require a shunt for optimal improvement of their headaches.

68. Is there a difficult shunt patient?

Unfortunately, this term is used to describe a group of patients who repeatedly visit the emergency room and have multiple surgeries for repeated shunt problems and malfunctions. Most of these patients are well known to the emergency room staff. Some of these patients have so called "slit ventricle syndrome" and present with headaches and repeated shunt malfunctions. These patients usually present a challenge to the neurosurgeon's clinical, technical, and social skills.

It has been my experience that no patient is really "a difficult shunt patient," and with patience and perseverance, all these patients can be managed effectively. It is highly essential to establish a rapport with the patient and the family at the earliest opportunity, which goes a long way in managing this group of patients.

It has been my experience that no patient is really "a difficult shunt patient," and with patience and perseverance, all these patients can be managed effectively.

PART FIFTEEN

Hydrocephalus, Shunts, and Pregnancy

Is hydrocephalus a contraindication for pregnancy?

I have a functioning shunt. Can amniocentesis be performed safely?

What precautions are required in the postpartum period in a patient with a shunt? Can a mother with a shunt breast-feed her newborn?

More...

With improved outcome of hydrocephalus, pregnancy in shunted women has become common. We will try to answer the commonly asked questions as per the current literature.

69. Is hydrocephalus a contraindication for pregnancy?

Obviously, the answer is no. With improved diagnosis and management, patients with hydrocephalus can be safely managed during pregnancy.

70. Do mothers with hydrocephalus have increased incidence of having children with birth defects? What is the role of prenatal testing in mothers with hydrocephalus? Does hydrocephalus predispose to an increased number of miscarriages?

Some studies reveal that mothers with hydrocephalus have a slightly higher incidence of children with birth defects. However, it is not definite for many reasons. To have a result with statistical significance, we need a large number of patients, and unfortunately, there are no randomized control studies of this circumstance. In addition, to complicate matters more, certain conditions associated with hydrocephalus or that cause hydrocephalus can be associated with increased risk of birth defects. For example, neural tube defects are known to be more common in subsequent pregnancies of mothers who have a child with spina bifida. Dandy-Walker malformations and neurofibromatosis are often hereditary, and presence of this condition in one sibling or in the parents indicates risk of increased birth defects. Some mothers are on long-term anticonvulsant medications, which may predispose them to have babies with birth defects or developmental deficits such as attention deficit disorder or autism. However, no studies suggest that the presence of shunts increase the risk of birth defects.

During pregnancy, prenatal testing of mothers with hydrocephalus is important to detect birth defects. Serial ultrasonography, serum alpha-fetoprotein, and amniocentesis in indicated cases have all been employed to detect birth defects. Until now, studies have not demonstrated any increased number of miscarriages with hydrocephalus or with the presence of shunts.

71. If investigations are required, can they be performed during pregnancy?

Of the available radiologic investigations, the important investigations that require consideration are X-ray, CT scan, and MRI scan. Both X-rays and CT scan involve radiation, and exposure to the fetus should be avoided if possible. MRI delivers a magnetic field and hence does not involve radiation exposure.

Radiation effects during pregnancy: The normal radiation exposure of the fetus is as follows:

> Abdominal X-ray: 0.1–0.3 rads
>
> Lumbar spine radiograph: 0.6 rads
>
> CT pelvis: 1–5 rads

These investigations, if needed, can be performed during pregnancy. However, risks and benefits of each should be considered.

The following is a brief summary of the available literature on the effects of radiation to the fetus (Bradley, 1998; Chen, 2008).

a.   **Spontaneous abortions** have been described with greater than 10 rad radiation dosage within 2 weeks of pregnancy. However, there is likely no increased risk if the embryo survives.

Hydrocephalus, Shunts, and Pregnancy

b. Between the 2nd and 20th week, the fetus is suscep-tible to *teratogenic effect of radiation.* This includes microcephaly, microphthalmia, mental retardation, growth restriction, cataracts, and behavioral defects. The threshold dosage to the fetus is around 5–15 rad. This is higher than the estimated radiation dosage from a maternal pelvic CT scan, which delivers ap-proximately between 2 and 4 rads, with the higher values toward the third trimester. Hence, teratogenic effect from a single pelvic CT scan is extremely un-likely.

c. There is always a risk of *carcinogenesis in the fetus* regardless of the dosage. Considering the available literature, it has been reported that a standard pelvic CT scan may increase the risk of fatal childhood cancer by up to twofold. Although the relative risk appears substantial, the baseline risk is considerably low (1 in 2,000), and it goes up to 2 in 2,000 after exposure of 5 rads. The risk also varies, depending on the trimester, with higher risks in the first trimes-ter (3.19) as compared with the second (1.29) and third trimesters (1.30). The 2004 guidelines of the American College of Obstetricians and Gynecolo-gists mentions that the carcinogenic risk of radiation during pregnancy is very small and abortion should not be recommended.

MRI in pregnancy: In general, most studies evaluating MRI during pregnancy show no ill effects. However, the current recommendation of the U.S. Food and Drug Administra-tion mentions that the safety of an MRI with respect to the fetus has not been established. The fetal concerns include (1) teratogenic effects and (2) acoustic effects.

Teratogenic effects: Although there have been some ani-mal studies indicating the possibility of teratogenic effects of MRI in early pregnancy, there have been no published human studies documenting ill effects of MRI on the fetus. With an exposure to 1.5 Tesla magnetic field, there have been no negative outcomes at 9 months and up to 9 years of age; there are no studies about exposure to higher magnetic field in pregnancy. However, in view of animal studies, sufficient caution is exercised, and the American College of Radiology guidance for safe MRI practices recommends that all pregnant patients can receive MRI as long as the risk–benefit ratio to the patient warrants that the study be performed. An MRI is presently considered a much safer option than any other imaging study involving ionizing radiation.

Acoustic effects: Although there is a theoretical possibility of acoustic damage to the fetus due to the exposure of loud noises generated by the MRI, no studies have found any significant correlation.

Contrast administration during pregnancy: Intravenous iodinated contrast agents (Iohexol) only should be used if absolutely necessary and only after informed consent is obtained. Iodinated contrast can induce hypothyroidism in the fetus though studies have demonstrated no effect of intravascular usage of nonionic contrast media on the fetus in inducing hypothyroidism.

During lactation, the standard recommendation is to discontinue breast-feeding for 24 hours after receiving intravascular iodinated contrast. However, recent articles conclude that iodinated contrast administration to breast-feeding women poses no risk to the infant and the previous recommendation is not indicated.

Gadolinium: Gadolinium is the contrast used in MRI scans. The U.S. Food and Drug Administration classifies gadolinium as Category C and recommends that it should not be used unless the requirement is considered critical. The risks and benefit of gadolinium should be explained to the patient.

72. I have a ventriculoperitoneal shunt and am pregnant. Should I be concerned about the functioning of the shunt? Do the shunts function adequately during pregnancy?

Because of the increasing size of the uterus during pregnancy, there are concerns regarding the functioning of ventriculoperitoneal shunts that use the abdominal cavity for CSF drainage. In the initial part of the pregnancy, there are no mechanical concerns to shunt malfunction. The uterus is relatively small and often does not cause any increase in intra-abdominal pressure. However, during the latter part of pregnancy, especially in the third trimester, patients often report significant headaches. This may result from increased size of the uterus resulting in increased intra-abdominal pressure.

Unfortunately, there is no single test to adequately evaluate and diagnose shunt failure. MRI has been used to monitor ventricular dilatation and may be considered rather than a CT scan, which exposes the fetus to radiation.

In rare cases, shunt catheters reportedly have disconnected and coiled around the reproductive organs during pregnancy. It is uncommon but has to be considered.

Studies have shown an increased frequency of ventriculo-peritoneal shunt malfunctions during or in the first 6 months after pregnancy compared with pregnant women with other shunts. This has been ascribed to several factors. First, studies have shown that CSF volume normally increases during pregnancy, being maximal at term. Second, there can be reduction in CSF drainage due to the increase volume of the uterus in the abdominal cavity. Further investigations are warranted to confirm these findings. However, all studies conclude that proper management of these patients can lead to normal pregnancy and delivery.

73. I have a functioning shunt. Can amniocentesis be performed safely?

Amniocentesis in indicated cases has been safely performed during pregnancy in patients with shunts. However, meticulous aseptic techniques should be used to minimize the risk of intraperitoneal infection.

74. Is it safe to have a normal delivery with a functioning shunt? Is cesarean section indicated in all patients with ventricular shunts?

Both vaginal delivery and cesarean section can be considered in patients with hydrocephalus and shunts. However, the proposed mode of delivery should consider the neurologic status of the patient, the relevant obstetric conditions, and the risks and benefits of the route for delivery. Neurologically asymptomatic or stable patients may be considered for vaginal delivery with a shortened second stage of labor. This avoids Valsalva efforts, which are frequent during the second stage of labor. Cesarean section is considered safe during pregnancy and can be used if normal delivery is not contemplated. However, cesarean section increases the risk of intra-abdominal infection and peritoneal scarring, which may jeopardize the shunt function, requiring its exteriorization or replacement.

There is no contraindication for administration of anesthesia either by epidural or spinal route. Special care should be taken to avoid infection and inadvertent drainage of CSF during the procedures.

Both vaginal delivery and cesarean section can be considered in patients with hydrocephalus and shunts.

75. What precautions are required in the postpartum period in a patient with a shunt? Can a mother with a shunt breast-feed her newborn?

Specifically, there are no extra precautions to be taken in the postpartum period. However, as discussed previously, shunt malfunctions for unknown reasons have been found to be slightly higher in the postpartum period than in the normal population. In addition, transient bacteremia, which is not uncommon postpartum, can induce shunt infections. Hence, if a systemic infection is suspected, broad-spectrum antibiotics should be started relatively early.

It is completely safe to breast-feed the child with a shunt.

76. If a shunt malfunctions during pregnancy, how it is best managed? Also, I would like to know more about endoscopic third ventriculostomy and its role in pregnancy.

Since symptoms suggesting shunt malfunction are common during a normal pregnancy, a conservative attitude is often initially practiced after a CT scan rules out ventricular enlargement. However, it is often difficult to generalize the approach, and each case should be considered on its own merit. If required, the peritoneal cavity may be avoided and a ventriculopleural or ventriculoatrial shunt maybe considered. Alternatively, endoscopic third ventriculostomy may also be considered if the patient is a suitable candidate.

Endoscopic third ventriculostomy may be considered as an alternative to shunt placement in indicated pregnant patients with hydrocephalus. This can be considered in both patients with newly diagnosed hydrocephalus who require surgery during pregnancy and in patients who have a shunt and present with shunt malfunction. Endoscopic third ventriculostomy avoids a laparotomy and does not require any special anesthesia. The efficacy of endoscopic third ventriculostomy in pregnant patients should be equivalent to the efficacy in the nonpregnant population of similar age group. Only a few reports in the literature indicate successful management of hydrocephalus in pregnancy with endoscopic third ventriculostomy and further studies would be required to assess the efficacy and any complications that may especially be associated with pregnancy.

PART SIXTEEN

Neuropsychologic Deficits in Hydrocephalus

My neurosurgeon asked for a neuropsychologic evaluation for my son during our last visit. Why is it required and when it is indicated?

What are the commonly used neuropsychologic tests?

What neuropsychologic deficits can be seen in infantile hydrocephalus?

77. My neurosurgeon asked for a neuropsychologic evaluation for my son during our last visit. Why is it required and when it is indicated?

In patients with hydrocephalus, a complete neurologic evaluation often reveals some degree of impairment of higher mental functions, such as memory, reasoning, and judgment. However, there has to be considerable impairment of these functions to be detected during a routine neurologic evaluation. Neuropsychologic evaluations, being more sensitive tests, can usually identify subtle deficits that are often missed during a neurologic evaluation.

It is very likely that a child with hydrocephalus will undergo neuropsychologic evaluation sometime during the initial few years. Under normal circumstances, a neuropsychologic evaluation is done during the follow-up of a patient with shunt. It is also performed in cooperative patients with chronic hydrocephalus in the preoperative period. This serves as a preoperative baseline evaluation, which is often helpful in assessing the benefits of the surgery by comparing with the postoperative evaluation. Neuropsychologic evaluation is also beneficial in ascertaining scholastic performance in the school-aged child. Pediatric neurosurgeons often request yearly or biannual assessments to identify subtle deficits that often can be managed by therapy or modifications in the school academic curriculum. In adults, a neuropsychologic evaluation is often indicated in assessing the overall cognitive impairment and for disability assessment purposes.

In the following questions, we will briefly discuss commonly performed neuropsychologic tests. We will also briefly enumerate various neuropsychologic defects that may be found in children with hydrocephalus. A detailed discussion is outside the scope of this book.

78. What are the commonly used neuropsychologic tests?

A variety of test batteries are currently used as neuropsychologic tests. These essentially are standardized tests that measure intelligence, learning and memory, visuospatial skills, fine-motor coordination, and attention and execution skills.

79. What neuropsychologic deficits can be seen in infantile hydrocephalus?

Several types of cognitive deficits can be associated with hydrocephalus. In the following pages, these are discussed under impairments of intelligence, motor skill, visuospatial skills, memory, language, executive functions, and behavior.

With a similar severity of hydrocephalus, it has been found that the deficits associated with congenital hydrocephalus are more extensive than with acquired hydrocephalus because early brain insults have more profound consequences than insults in later childhood.

Intelligence: Congenital or acquired hydrocephalus in children can affect intelligence. Overall intelligence has been reported to be low average or below average in hydrocephalic children. However, in the past few decades, with more and more children undergoing shunt insertion early in life, the degree of impaired intelligence has improved considerably. In children with hydrocephalus, some studies show that verbal intelligence is relatively more affected than nonverbal intelligence. Several studies have shown that the level of intelligence has been related to the degree of hydrocephalus, the degree of myelination of the brain, the ventricular size and thickness of the cortical mantle before and after shunting, and the occurrence of complications and secondary injury to the brain. This is evidenced by significant impairment of intelligence quotient (IQ) in conditions causing secondary brain insults as in children with associated intraventricular hemorrhage, asphyxia, and shunt infections. However, number and frequency of shunt revisions do not significantly affect IQ.

Motor skills: Motor deficits range widely from fine-motor impairment in the upper limbs to gross-walking disturbances. Children with associated brain or spinal cord injury demonstrate additional motor dysfunctions consistent with the location of the lesion. For example, children with myelomeningocele have associated lower-limb weakness while those with neonatal intraventricular hemorrhage have spastic weakness of the lower limbs (cerebral palsy). There is a relative preponderance of left-handedness in children with hydrocephalus as compared with the general population (the incidence ranges between 22% and 40%). In some studies of children with spina bifida and hydrocephalus, left-handedness has correlated with poor performance in motor measures and was related to the preoperative severity of hydrocephalus. In addition, motor planning has also been found to be impaired in hydrocephalic children.

Visuospatial skills: Visuospatial skills are consistently reduced in children with hydrocephalus. Reduction in visuospatial skills commonly correlates with a predominant dilatation of the occipital horns and posterior part of the lateral ventricle. It has been suggested that this may be related to the anomalies of the splenium of corpus callosum (the posterior part of a large band of fibers that connects both halves of the brain and forms the roof of the lateral ventricles) seen predominantly in hydrocephalic children.

Memory: Memory impairments are a common complaint in older children with hydrocephalus. It is, however, possible that impaired attention and retrieval may be partly responsible for the impaired memory. Of the several areas of the brain known to be responsible for memory, the anterior temporal neocortex is essential for long-term memory storage. The hippocampus is the primary area for transfer of short-term memory information into long-term storage. As the white matter tracts conveying impulses to and from the hippocampus are located near the lateral and third ventricles, the effect of ventricular dilatation can stretch and impair functioning of these fibers. Although several studies have been performed, consistent results in the type and pattern of memory deficits in hydrocephalus have not been well established. Memory impairment also has been suggested to be partly responsible for learning impairment often seen in these children.

Language skills: Although there is no global impairment of language functions in hydrocephalus, hydrocephalic children appear to be less skilled as compared with their peers. *Receptive language* skill impairments have been found to be deficiencies in understanding written language and sometimes spoken language. There may be impairment of passage comprehension and in the ability to produce antonyms and synonyms. In *productive language*, these children are usually fluent and verbose. However, often they lack coherence, which is well brought out in storytelling. There may also be deficiencies of structured sentence generation.

A specific type of language pattern known as *cocktail party syndrome* has been identified in hydrocephalic children. This is characterized by fluent and well-articulated speech, vocabulary above the apparent mental level of functioning but with shallow intellect and poor social and academic skills. There is usually excessive use of stereotyped phrases and verbal perseveration. It has been reported that cocktail party syndrome may be seen in 28–40% of children with spina bifida and hydrocephalus.

Executive functions: Executive functions are often difficult to assess, as they are closely related to attention and memory functions. It is commonly believed that such functions as concept formation, flexibility, and planning are mediated by the prefrontal cortex. This is manifested by poor scores on the Wisconsin Card Sorting Test (used to test preservative errors and mental flexibility) and on the Tower of London test (which tests planning abilities).

Behavior and social functions: With the limited available data, children with hydrocephalus have been described to have increased incidence of social and behavioral difficulties. In prior studies, up to two-thirds of children with hydrocephalus were reported to have significant behavioral problems. However, most children with hydrocephalus mentioned their family relationships to be good despite extreme emotional, financial, and physical stresses associated with hydrocephalus.

Academic achievement and school performance: About 60% of children with shunted hydrocephalus have been reported to attend regular classes. However, of these, about half lag behind their normal age peers in school by 1–2 years. Low arithmetic scores have been reported in hydrocephalic children, while their reading abilities have been found to be within normal range.

School placement and achievement level has been found to be significantly related to the etiology of hydrocephalus. Twenty-nine percent of children with congenital hydrocephalus attended special schools, while the percentage was higher in those with acquired etiologies, such as meningitis (52%) and intraventricular hemorrhage (60%).

PART SEVENTEEN

Intraventricular Hemorrhage of the Newborn

What is intraventricular hemorrhage of a newborn?
What is the cause of the bleeding? How severe can
the bleeding be?

What investigations are required? How is the
hydrocephalus managed?

What is the outcome? Can the intraventricular
hemorrhage be prevented?

More...

80. What is intraventricular hemorrhage of a newborn? What is the cause of the bleeding? How severe can the bleeding be?

This is another common cause of secondary hydrocephalus in newborns. It is most common in infants less than 32 weeks of gestation and is often seen in infants 35 weeks or less. Many of the hemorrhages are asymptomatic and detected in routine neonatal ultrasound evaluation. For this reason, it is difficult to assess the overall incidence of neonatal intraventricular hemorrhage (IVH). However, the overall incidence may be as high as 40–45% of prematurely born babies who weigh less than 1,500 grams or are less than 35 weeks of gestation.

Most IVH occur early after birth with about 50% of neonatal IVH occuring within 24 hours of birth and 90% by the end of third day of life. In about one-fifth cases, hemorrhage can actually progress.

Cause of bleeding: In the premature infant, walls of the blood vessels in the region of germinal matrix (located in the wall of the lateral ventricle near its external angle, near the head of caudate nucleus) lack the necessary structural elements that often give stability to the vessels in adults. These blood vessels involute around 32–34 weeks of gestational age. Normally, these vessels are not exposed to the fluctuations in the blood pressure while the fetus is in the uterus. However, in prematurely born infants (before these blood vessels involute), these fragile blood vessels are exposed to arterial and venous pressure surges and rupture, causing intraventricular hemorrhage. In severe cases, associated intraparenchymal hemorrhage usually occurs.

Severity of the bleeding: Severity of the hemorrhage is separated into four grades:

- Grade I: germinal matrix hemorrhage without extension into the ventricle
- Grade II: intraventricular hemorrhage involving up to 50% of the ventricular area, no ventricular dilatation

- Grade III: intraventricular hemorrhage involving 50% or more ventricular area, associated ventricular dilatation
- Grade IV: intraventricular hemorrhage with associated intraparenchymal hemorrhage

Following the bleeding, three significant pathological changes may occur: (1) periventricular hemorrhagic infarctions, (2) development of hydrocephalus, and (3) development of periventricular leukomalacia.

In periventricular hemorrhagic infarction, due to the obstruction to the draining veins by the germinal matrix hemorrhage, adjacent white matter has stasis of blood and becomes infarcted (hemorrhagic infarction). It occurs in around 15% of infants. Usually, it occurs on one side of the brain, though in a third of patients, it can occur on both sides.

Hydrocephalus develops in these children by the clot obstructing the CSF pathways either in the ventricular system (third ventricle, aqueduct, fourth ventricle) or outside the ventricular system (arachnoid granulations, subarachnoid spaces). As there may be a lag of several days to weeks between identifying the hemorrhage and the subsequent development of ventricular dilatation, it may be related to the breakdown of the blood products that cause hydrocephalus.

In addition, whiter matter injury around the ventricles, known as periventricular leukomalacia, can develop. This is believed to be due to decreased blood supply to the surrounding white brain matter, thus leading to infarction.

As we will see later, these three significantly influence mortality, morbidity, and overall long-term outcome.

81. How do these present? Why do these children develop hydrocephalus?

The presentation is either acute, subacute, or asymptomatic. In the acute presentation, there may be deterioration in neurologic status, change in muscle tone, seizures, or respiratory or cardiac irregularities. Usually, this is associated with a tense fontanel and a drop in hematocrit (hemoglobin level in blood) by 10% or more. In subacute presentation, gradual fullness of fontanel, irritability, and reduced motor activity may be the presenting symptoms.

About 20–50% of infants with germinal matrix hemorrhage will ultimately develop either transient or progressive hydrocephalus. The higher grades (Grades III and IV) will have higher incidences of hydrocephalus than the lower grades (Grades I and II). As mentioned earlier, most of the time the hydrocephalus appears 1 to three 3 after the hemorrhage. Developing hydrocephalus usually manifests by abnormal increase in the head circumference, lethargy, bradycardia (low heart rate) with worsening respiratory efforts, and inability to maintain oxygen saturations.

The incidence of development of hydrocephalus has been found to be directly related to the grade of intraventricular hemorrhage. Approximately 5% of Grade I, 20% of Grade II, 55% of Grade III, and 80% of Grade IV will develop ventriculomegaly (Volpe, 1989). Among the survivors, ultimately 60% will require shunt insertion, with the incidence being higher in the higher grades.

82. What investigations are required? How is the hydrocephalus managed?

Taking advantage of the open fontanel, cranial ultrasound evaluations can diagnose the intracranial hemorrhage fairly easily (**Figure 38**). In addition, they are quick, noninvasive, and do not involve radiation to the newborn. Most important, the procedure is performed at the bedside, thus the sick infant does not have to be transported. Head ultrasounds are usually repeated twice a week to assess for hematoma resolution, development of hydrocephalus, or occurrence of new hemorrhage. CT scan or MRI is sometimes performed before shunt placement.

About 20–50% of infants with germinal matrix hemorrhage will ultimately develop either transient or progressive hydrocephalus. The higher grades (Grades III and IV) will have higher incidences of hydrocephalus than the lower grades (Grades I and II).

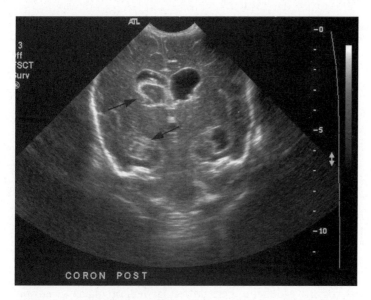

Figure 38. Cranial Ultrasound Demonstrating Intraventricular Hemorrhage in a Newborn. (Arrows)

Management: Apart from overall management, development of hydrocephalus warrants measures to drain the CSF externally for the initial few weeks. This is because of several considerations. Initially, the blood-mixed CSF makes the shunt placement unsuitable, as blood can obstruct the shunt pathways. There is also a higher incidence of shunt infection in premature babies as compared with term babies. In addition, the child may be too unstable to undergo the shunt procedure, as several systemic conditions (respiratory distress syndrome, septicemia) are known to occur during this period. Last, not every infant with neonatal intraventricular hemorrhage would require a shunt insertion as in certain percentages of cases; the hydrocephalus spontaneously resolves or resolves after intermittent ventricular taps.

The CSF drainage is usually performed either by intermittent percutaneous ventricular taps, placement of external drain, or placement of a reservoir and intermittent reservoir taps. The status of hydrocephalus is usually monitored with intermittent cranial ultrasounds. If the child requires permanent CSF drainage, a ventriculoperitoneal shunt is considered once the CSF becomes clear and the overall clinical condition is stable. Usually, most neurosurgeons wait until the child reaches the term age or weighs 2,000 grams or more.

83. What is the outcome? Can the intraventricular hemorrhage be prevented?

Infants with neonatal IVH have a higher mortality rate (16–35%) as compared with premature infants without IVH (6.5–13%). Overall mortality and morbidity risk depend on the grade of IVH, associated periventricular hemorrhagic infarction, and periventricular leukomalacia. Periventricular hemorrhagic infarction most commonly results in hemiparesis, which affects predominantly the lower extremities as well as cognitive deficits. Periventricular leukomalacia usually is responsible for spastic diplegia (stiffness of the lower extremities) due to injury to the descending white matter tracts from the leg area of the motor cortex to the spinal cord. Children with hydrocephalus requiring a shunt fare worse than those who do not require shunt.

It has been reported that of 5% in Grade I, 10% in Grade II, 20% in Grade III, and 50% with Grade IV hemorrhage will ultimately not survive. Similarly, it was found that the permanent neurologic deficits for patients with Grade I IVH was 5%, Grade II was 15%, Grade III was 35%, and Grade IV was 90%.

Regarding prevention of intraventricular hemorrhage, of the several medications that have been tried, recent studies indicate early postnatal low-dose indomethacin may reduce the incidence of neonatal IVH and development of parenchyma insult to the developing brain.

PART EIGHTEEN

Benign External Hydrocephalus

What is benign external hydrocephalus? Why does it happen?

How does it present?

How is it diagnosed?

More...

84. What is benign external hydrocephalus? Why does it happen?

This is a condition exclusively seen in children. It is also known by several other names: subdural hygroma in infancy, benign expansion of subarachnoid spaces, and benign frontal extracerebral fluid collection of infancy. We will use the term *benign external hydrocephalus* for purposes of this discussion. Although some consider the term *hydrocephalus* a misnomer in this condition, in real terminologies, it is not, if we realize that the term hydrocephalus denotes excessive accumulation of CSF in the intracranial compartment, which is true to a certain extent in the present circumstances.

Although the cause is uncertain, it has been suggested that a relative immaturity of the arachnoid villi fails to absorb the required amount of CSF into the bloodstream. With the obstruction at the level of the arachnoid villi, a communicating type of hydrocephalus develops, with CSF accumulating in both the ventricular system and the subarachnoid spaces.

85. How does it present?

This condition is almost exclusively reserved for infants and young children who are between 6 and 12 months of age and invariably younger than age 24 months. The presentation is usually a child who has a slightly larger head for his or her age group. The head circumference when plotted in the head circumference curve measures either or near the 95th or 98th percentile and in most circumstances follows the curve. The anterior fontanel usually remains open for a longer period before it closes, though it remains soft and lax. The open anterior fontanel along with the relatively larger head raises concern from the pediatrician, and a CT scan is performed to rule out hydrocephalus.

The child's developmental status may reveal a mild delay in overall gross-motor and cognitive development. The delay may not be more than few months lag from the child's peers and manifests more in motor than in cognitive aspects.

86. How is it diagnosed?

The CT or the MRI scan usually reveals evidence of a prominent ventricular system that is larger than the normal range, with prominent subarachnoid spaces (**Figure 39**). Fluid in the subarachnoid space does not appear to exert compression on the underlying brain parenchyma, which appears relaxed and uncompromised. Presence of gross ventriculomegaly usually rules out a diagnosis of benign external hydrocephalus. The brain parenchyma appears otherwise normal.

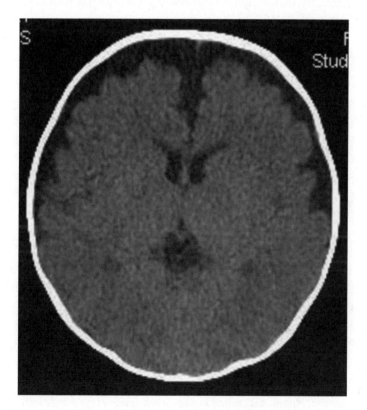

Figure 39. CT Scan of Benign External Hydrocephalus. Note the extra CSF on the surface of the brain with mildly prominent ventricles.

It is essential that we rule out some other conditions that can mimic benign external hydrocephalus. In *subdural hygroma*, there is accumulation in the CSF in the subdural space which causes compression on the underlying brain parenchyma by obliterating the sulci (clefts seen on the surface of brain). Also the fluid in subdural hygroma is slightly more proteinaceous and appears different in MRI than the CSF in benign external hydrocephalus. *Cerebral atrophy* in children can also present as prominent subarachnoid spaces in the CT and MRI scans. However, the fluid collection is seen equally distributed both anteriorly and posteriorly over the surface of the brain unlike in external hydrocephalus, where fluid is seen predominantly anteriorly. In addition, children with brain atrophy should not have a relatively large head.

87. Does it need treatment?

Mostly, this is a self-limiting condition and self-corrects within 2 years time.

Mostly, this is a self-limiting condition and self-corrects within 2 years time. The head circumference continues to stay along the 95th percentile but parallels the growth curve without off-shooting and slowly joins the curve around 2 years time. The child continues to develop motor and cognitive skills and compares well with peers. It is essential to reassure the family and evaluate the head circumference so that it stays parallel to the curve over the next few months.

Infrequently, head circumference grows disproportionately and shoots up in the head circumference curve. In such cases, placement of a subduroperitoneal shunt may be considered, predominantly to arrest the increase in head circumference. Often, these shunts are not required after 2–3 years of age and may be removed.

Gillian's comment:

Our son, Adam, was noted to have a relatively large head around 6 months of age, noted during a routine clinic checkup. We searched the Internet and got worried, knowing that it could be something as severe to require a surgery. The CT scan done showed some extra fluid on the surface of the brain. When we saw the neurosurgeon, he mentioned it was a condition known as benign external hydrocephalus. He explained to us about it and indicated that most children would not require any surgery. The head growth stabilized over the next few months. We took Adam every 3 months for a checkup. Now at 2 years of age, he has a slightly larger head than his peers. Otherwise, he is a happy toddler.

Benign External Hydrocephalus

PART NINETEEN

Normal Pressure Hydrocephalus

What is normal pressure hydrocephalus?

What investigations are indicated once a diagnosis is made?

What surgical procedures are considered for normal pressure hydrocephalus?

More...

88. What is normal pressure hydrocephalus?

Normal pressure hydrocephalus (NPH) is a type of communicating hydrocephalus encountered mostly in elderly persons. There is excessive accumulation of the CSF in the intracranial compartment with dilatation of ventricles and the subarachnoid spaces. The clinical picture is classical of an elderly patient, who presents with the triad of gait ataxia, dementia, and urinary incontinence. It is important to recognize normal pressure hydrocephalus early because it is a form of *treatable dementia*, and if treated successfully, it can be significantly improved, if not completely reversed. Unfortunately, most patients with normal pressure hydrocephalus are either underdiagnosed or misdiagnosed in clinical practice. This is because all patients do not present with the classical triad of gait ataxia, dementia, and incontinence. Most commonly they have one or two of the above symptoms. In addition, most of these symptoms, individually or together, can be present in this age group because of other diagnoses. For example, prostatic hypertrophy is commonly seen in elderly males and can be thought of as causing urinary symptoms; arthritis can be considered responsible for slow walking, and senile dementia may be responsible for memory impairment. It common to have one or more of these conditions in the elderly age group, and an associated normal pressure hydrocephalus can be missed because of these overlapping coexistent conditions. Another factor that possibly delays effective treatment is the reluctance to consider shunt procedures in this age group. Delaying the definitive treatment considerably reduces chances of overall improvement. While evaluating an elderly patient consider the existence of normal pressure hydrocephalus and pay attention to identifying the condition at an early stage.

It is important to recognize normal pressure hydrocephalus early because it is a form of treatable dementia, and if treated successfully, it can be significantly improved, if not completely reversed.

89. Why do some people develop normal pressure hydrocephalus? How frequently is this seen in the general population?

As originally described in 1965, this condition was considered to be *idiopathic* (cause relatively unknown). Over the next 40 years, though we know more about this condition, we still do not know what causes CSF to accumulate. It is thought that the arachnoid granulations "age," leading to decreased CSF absorption. Slow insidious insults may cause scarring of the subarachnoid spaces and granulations. In patients with normal pressure hydrocephalus, the brain parenchyma is less stiff (more compliant) to allow for it to be compressed by the developing ventriculomegaly and thus does not result in increased intracranial pressure. However, this is not always true, as intermittent increases in intracranial pressures have been detected by several investigators.

In subsequent years, it has been found that hydrocephalus developing after several primary insults can present as normal pressure hydrocephalus. The notable example of this is chronic posttraumatic hydrocephalus that results after severe head injury. Other conditions that can mimic idiopathic normal pressure hydrocephalus are posthemorrhagic hydrocephalus, hydrocephalus following meningitis, and hydrocephalus after previous neurosurgical intervention. Not uncommonly, one sees a chronic, slowly developing obstructive hydrocephalus mimicking as normal pressure hydrocephalus.

It is often difficult to assess the overall incidence of normal pressure hydrocephalus. However, some studies report an overall incidence of 2–20 per million per year in the population. Its incidence is higher among assisted care living and nursing home populations. A recent report revealed that 9–14% of patients may be diagnosed as NPH, considering the criteria used for diagnosis (Marmarou 2005).

Normal Pressure Hydrocephalus

90. How do these patients present?

The classic picture is that of the elderly person presenting with gait abnormality, memory impairment, and incontinence. We will elaborate on these symptoms in detail.

Gait abnormality: This is often the earliest symptom and manifests as a shuffling gait with a relatively widened base. Some call it a magnetic gait, as the feet appear to be stuck to the ground, and the patient has difficulty lifting his or her feet. There may be also difficulty turning corners while walking with a tendency to fall. Typically, there is no significant associated weakness in the legs. The overall gait appears as diminished ability to move smoothly.

Cognitive deficits: Cognitive impairment is manifested by forgetfulness and generalized slowness of thought. These are usually gradual and are not as severe as in Alzheimer's disease. Memory dysfunction may affect recent events and is associated with verbal dysfluency and planning defects. There may be associated behavioral disturbances, agitation, and delusions, though these are uncommon.

Urinary disturbances: Urinary disturbances in normal pressure hydrocephalus result in increased frequency and urgency. In later stages, it may be associated with incontinence. In addition, the associated slow gait can hinder early access to the toilet and thus add to the problem. Some patients in late stage may be unable to realize the need to urinate and thus may wet their pants. Rarely fecal incontinence is encountered.

Of the three symptoms, classically the gait difficulty is the earliest to appear, followed by memory impairment and then urinary incontinence.

Patients with normal pressure hydrocephalus usually do not have seizures, numbness, weakness, and speech disturbances other than those mentioned, nor do they have other focal deficits. However, other neurologic conditions can coexist in this age group, and the previous symptoms may be associated because of these coexistent conditions.

91. What investigations are indicated once a diagnosis is made?

Unfortunately, there is no single investigation that can diagnose or rule out this condition. We will briefly discuss various investigations currently available.

CT and MRI: CT and MRI scans show dilatation of all the ventricles and prominent subarachnoid spaces, suggesting a communicating hydrocephalus. The ventricular enlargement is usually out of proportion to the sulcal prominence, which is a key finding in distinguishing brain atrophy, which is commonly seen in this age group. The MRI scan is particularly beneficial to rule out insidious aqueductal stenosis, which can often present with slow development of hydrocephalus and normal pressure hydrocephalus–like symptoms. This is important because with the current recommendations patients with aqueductal stenosis are considered to be ideal candidates for an endoscopic CSF diversion procedure that makes them shunt independent.

There has not been a single finding that proves the diagnosis. The CT or MRI report would often read "ventricular enlargement which is consistent with the patient's age. However, normal pressure hydrocephalus cannot be ruled out and clinical correlation is required." Probably, the most important aspect of these investigations is to exclude causes that can present like multi-infarct dementia or, in certain cases, a slowly progressing brain tumor.

Cisternography: Cisternography has been commonly used in the past to diagnose NPH. However, like previous tests, results of the test are not specific for the condition. Normally,

Cisternography

A radiological study in which a contrast or a dye is placed in the cisterns by a spinal tap to study the flow of the cerebrospinal fluid.

a spinal tap is performed and a radioactive isotope is injected into the subarachnoid space. The images are then obtained at 3, 6, and 24 hours after injection to assess the distribution of the isotope. Normally, 24 hours after injection, radioactivity is symmetrically distributed over the cerebral convexities without any intraventricular accumulation. In some normal persons, there may be some intraventricular accumulation in the first 24 hours but not after. In normal pressure hydrocephalus, there is early activity in the ventricles with persistent of activity after 24 hours. This is thought due to reflux of the isotope into the ventricular system due to its relative nonabsorption from the arachnoid granulations.

Cisternography has been found to be far from diagnosing normal pressure hydrocephalus, and currently, it is believed that this technique is no more sensitive than clinical assessment and does not predict response to treatment.

Therapeutic trial of CSF drainage: Therapeutic trial of CSF drainage has been used in patients suspected of normal pressure hydrocephalus to predict response to treatment. Two forms of this procedure are currently in practice: (a) high volume intermittent lumbar puncture and CSF drainage (b) placement of an external lumbar drain.

a. **High volume intermittent lumbar puncture:** This commonly involves performing lumbar puncture on an outpatient basis and removing around 30 cubic centimeters of CSF. Recent studies, however, have suggested that up to 50 cubic centimeters of CSF may be removed for higher sensitivity. Usually, the family is asked to report any improvement in gait and memory functions. Although only a limited CSF is removed during the procedure, there is a small amount of persistent CSF leak into the epidural space, which persists for a few days after the spinal tap. In patients who do not improve, some may consider repeating this procedure for a consecutive 3 or

4 days to see whether there is any improvement. Accuracy for this test in predicting a favorable outcome from surgery varies between 45% and 54%.

b. **Placement of continuous lumbar drain:** For this, the patient is admitted to the hospital and an external lumbar drain is placed and connected to a bag that connects the spinal fluid. A limited predetermined amount of CSF (usually 10 cubic centimeters per hour) is drained for the next few days and any improvement in the patients overall status is assessed. The accuracy of this test in predicting a favorable outcome from shunt varies between 58% and 100%.

Of the two procedures, extended CSF drainage with placement of a lumbar drain has higher accuracy in identifying patients who would benefit from the procedure. This indicates that a significant number of patients who do not improve with a large volume lumbar puncture will still improve with prolonged drainage and benefit from shunting. There is a common belief that many patients who do not improve after a spinal tap and CSF drainage will not benefit from surgery. In fact, some neurologists do not refer patients to the neurosurgeon unless they have improved following the drainage of CSF. However, studies have also shown that a significant group of patients benefit from shunt surgery even if there was no significant improvement following high-volume CSF drainage. In a previous study, as high as 65% of patients who did not benefit either after the lumbar puncture and drainage or after placement of external ventricular drain ultimately improved after placement of a shunt (Walchenbach, 2002). This is why some consider that the ultimate therapeutic trial may be shunt surgery. However, this approach may be associated with higher overall failures, as patients who would not have satisfied the criteria for surgery are included. In addition, it may not be prudent to consider patients for surgical procedures in which there have been associated risks. All these indicate that a thorough clinical evaluation is essential in arriving at the diagnosis.

Estimation of CSF outflow resistance (also known as CSF impedance or Ro): This is a relatively recent area of investigation to identify patients who would benefit from the shunt procedure. The Ro of CSF is considered to be the impedance of flow offered by the CSF absorption pathways. Conductance is the reciprocal of resistance. Both conductance and impedance are used in various studies, and there is no significant preference among investigators about which term should predominate as both give similar information.

To estimate Ro, artificial CSF is introduced into the lumbar subarachnoid space at a known rate by a lumbar puncture. The Ro is calculated by estimating the difference between the final steady pressure reached and the initial pressure divided by the rate of infusion.

Although there have been several studies of establishing the relationship of Ro with the likelihood of improvement after surgery, there still is no consensus regarding the accuracy of Ro predicting the outcome after shunt surgery. The reported accuracy for improvement after the surgery varies from 54% to 96%. No doubt this is higher than the lumbar puncture and CSF drainage test, but we still need to have more studies to recommend its routine clinical usage.

Aqueductal CSF Flow in MRI: There have been some studies demonstrating that patients of NPH who may ultimately improve with shunt surgery have higher CSF flow velocity through the aqueduct. However, other studies have not revealed a correlation between the CSF flows though the aqueduct and responsiveness to shunting. However, further studies are required before a conclusion can be reached. The only advantage is that unlike other procedures, this is noninvasive and has no complications.

92. What surgical procedures are considered for normal pressure hydrocephalus?

Of the various surgical procedures currently recommended, drainage of CSF from the ventricular cavity by ventriculo-peritoneal or ventriculoatrial shunt is commonly considered. Drainage of CSF from the lumbar subarachnoid space by lumboperitoneal shunt has also been considered but is not currently widely practiced. The role of endoscopic third ven-triculostomy has been controversial with some initial studies demonstrating success; however, subsequent studies have not substantiated that success.

Of all these surgical procedures, there is a high degree of unanimity choosing the procedure for the ventriculoperito-neal shunts. However, there has been variability in choosing the exact type of shunt composition and valve specification for insertion. We will briefly enumerate the various types of shunt composition that can be used for treating normal pres-sure hydrocephalus.

Type of valve: fixed pressure versus programmable valve versus flow-regulated valve: As discussed in the previous chapter, there are basically two broad categories of shunt valves: pressure regulated and flow regulated.

Pressure-regulated valves open at a certain pressure setting, while flow-regulated valves drain CSF at a constant flow rate. Both types of valves have been used for normal pres-sure hydrocephalus. Pressure-controlled valves are either *fixed pressure* or are variable pressure setting (programmable). The advantages of *programmable valves* are that the pressure setting can be adjusted between a range 3 centimeters of CSF to 20 centimeters of CSF pressure with an external magnetic device. Thus, in many cases, either underdrainage or overdrainage can be managed nonsurgically by adjusting the pressure setting in the valve appropriately. In fixed pressure valves, the patient would need another surgical procedure to replace the valve.

One study demonstrated that on an average eight adjustments were required for each patient. Of these, 24% were for overdrainage, 54% for underdrainage, and 9% were considered for subdural collections. Of these, approximately 50% of the valve adjustments were thought to be clinically beneficial. There are currently several adjustable valves available; notable among them are the Codman Hakim programmable valve, Medtronic PS Medical Strata programmable valve, Polaris programmable valve and Aesculap-Miethke proGav.

Some patients with fixed pressure valves will overdrain by siphoning, thus requiring antisiphon devices apart from adjusting their valves. Antisiphon devices retard the flow of the CSF when the patient is in an upright position and hence prevents sudden and excessive drainage of fluid with change in body position. Some neurosurgeons incorporate antisiphon devices in all patients with normal pressure hydrocephalus while others will add them only if required.

Flow-regulated valves limit CSF flow by allowing only a limited amount of CSF under normal conditions and automatically switch to a high flow rate under conditions of increased intracranial pressure. The examples of the flow regulated valve are the Orbis Sigma valve (Integra) and the Phoenix Diamond valves (Vygon Neuro). The greatest advantages of the flow-regulated valves are that overdrainage from siphoning is prevented in most cases, though an occasional overdrainage and subdural hematoma formation has been reported.

Which is the optimal valve? A previous study comparing the efficacy of programmable valves and flow-regulated valves did not find any significant advantage of one type of valve over another. Programmable valves have definite advantage over nonprogrammable fixed pressure valves in optimizing the ideal pressure setting for an individual patient and in reducing the number of potential surgeries after insertion. Universal inclusion of antisiphon devices is probably not recommended, as it would considerably reduce the drainage, thus limiting overall outcome in a group of patients despite a low opening pressure setting in the valve.

Lumboperitoneal shunt: Lumboperitoneal shunts have been often used as the initial surgical option in normal pressure hydrocephalus. However, most indications have been for patients in whom ventricular shunts are contraindicated. Though simpler, these are not very popular among neurosurgeons because of lack of availability of good lumbar valve systems along with the occurrence of increased mechanical malfunctions as compared with ventricular shunts.

Subdural collection and hemorrhage: The most concerning complication of shunts in normal pressure hydrocephalus has been the development of subdural collections. Subdural collections can be subdural effusions (hygroma) and subdural hematoma. The basic difference between the two is that the fluid is usually watery and nonbloody, although the fluid may be slightly yellowish in the former, while it is usually either liquefied or clotted blood in the latter. The incidence of subdural effusions has varied between 2% and 17%.

Subdural collections often occur following the release of CSF as the ventricular cavity reduces in size and the brain parenchyma does not expand adequately to fill up the space. However, the brain parenchyma often collapses and creates a subdural space (**Figure 40**). The veins that normally traverse between the brain and the dura get stretched and may rupture or have small tears in their walls from which the blood leaks and accumulates in the preformed subdual space. Most of the time the bleeding spontaneously subsides and the condition remains asymptomatic until diagnosed by a routine follow-up CT scan. However, not uncommonly the bleeding can be significant to cause worsening in neurologic symptoms. In patients on anticoagulants or antiplatelet agents it often can be devastating, requiring urgent surgical evacuation.

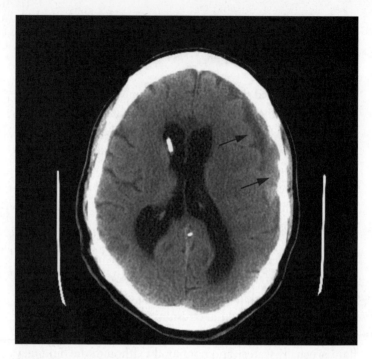

Figure 40. CT Scan with Left Subdural Collection with Bleeding in a Pateint with NPH. (Arrows)

Small subdural effusions will not often require surgical intervention and can be safely observed. However, larger subdural collections will require evacuation. Often, mild to moderate subdural collections can be effectively managed by raising the shunt valve pressure, which essentially reduces the CSF drainage, dilates the ventricular system, and consequently reduces the subdural space. In some cases with overdrainage predominantly due to siphoning, insertion of an antisiphon device would be required (**Figure 41**). However, both raising the pressure setting in the programmable valve and inserting an antisiphon device reduce the overall CSF outflow from the ventricles, which may lead to the recurrence of initial presurgery symptoms.

Apart from development of subdural collections, other shunt complications that can occur include infection, malfunction,

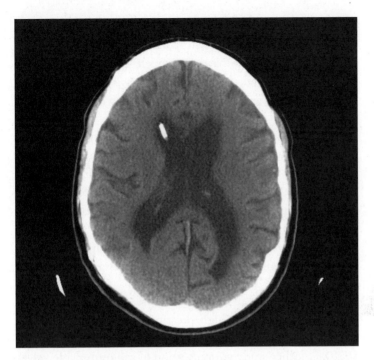

Figure 41. Resolution of the Subdural Collection in the Same Patient with Reprogramming of the Shunt.

intracranial bleeding such as intracerebral hematoma, or seizures. These risks are similar to the normal population, though the risk of intracerebral bleeding may be higher, as most patients may be on antiplatelet agents or anticoagulants.

93. What is the prognosis and the natural history of normal pressure hydrocephalus? How favorable is the outcome?

Several studies have shown that an early diagnosis and treatment has higher success rates than a late diagnosis. Patients with less than 6 months of symptoms have the highest chances of improvement, while those with symptoms, particularly dementia, present for more than 2 or 3 years have lower rates of improvement. Also, it has been proven that patients who have *one or two symptoms* of the classical triad have a better prognosis

Several studies have shown that an early diagnosis and treatment has higher success rates than a late diagnosis.

for improvement than those who have a complete triad. Hence, patients either with gait disturbances or dementia improve better than those who have a complete triad. Of the various components of triad, patients *presenting with gait disturbances* improve more often than those presenting with dementia.

The favorable predictors for outcome have been an early appearance of gait disorder, shorter duration of symptoms, clinical response to CSF removal by drainage lumbar puncture or drain, and high resistance of CSF infusion test. Similarly, the unfavorable outcome predictors can be summarized as early appearance of dementia, dementia present for more than 2 years, absence of gait disorder or appearing after dementia, and relative nonresponse to lumbar spinal drainage.

In a previous study, an improvement was noted in 53% of patients with medium- or high-pressure valves, whereas patients with low-pressure valves had a 74% improvement (Boon, 1998). Another study with insertion of programmable valves in 147 patients of normal pressure hydrocephalus had a good outcome reported in 90% of cases (Zemack and Romner, 2002).

Over several years of follow-up, studies have noted that the initial improvement usually reduces in a significant percentage of patients. The initial improvement of 64% at 3 months reduced to 26% at 3 years follow-up (Malm, 2000). Reduction in all aspects of improvement over 5 years as compared with 1 year was reported in another study. Gait disturbances reduced from 76% to 47%, memory improvement from 48% to 38%, and improvement in urinary incontinence from 58% to 29% (Savolainen, 2002).

In patients who deteriorate following initial improvement, shunt malfunction or underdrainage should be considered. However, with relatively large ventricles in these patients, proximal shunt obstruction is less likely. Under such circumstances, CSF underdrainage should be a strong concern, and the valve may be considered to be reprogrammed to a lower pressure if feasible. Improvement following a shunt tap or temporary drainage of CSF may indicate the diagnosis in such cases.

PART TWENTY

Idiopathic Intracranial Hypertension

What is idiopathic intracranial hypertension? What is the cause? Are there any predisposing factors?

How is the diagnosis confirmed?

What are the management options?

More...

94. What is idiopathic intracranial hypertension? What is the cause? Are there any predisposing factors?

The condition of chronic raised intracranial pressure without evidence of any mass lesion or ventriculomegaly has been known under a variety of terminologies. Of these, benign intracranial hypertension (BIH), idiopathic intracranial hypertension, and pseudotumor cerebri are the most commonly used. In this chapter, we will address the condition as **idiopathic intracranial hypertension (IIH)**. However, unlike the often used "benign" suggests, we should realize that in some patients this condition is far from benign and if not treated adequately can lead to permanent visual loss.

Idiopathic intracranial hypertension (IIH)

Also known as benign intracranial hypertension (BIH) or pseudotumor cerebri (PTC), this is a condition characterized by increased intracranial pressure in the absence of a tumor or other conditions such as hydrocephalus.

Although this condition is most often seen in obese young females, it is encountered in nonobese patients and even in males. The **diagnostic criteria** includes signs and symptoms of increased intracranial pressure, no neurologic deficits except for a VIth nerve paresis, normal to small ventricles in radiologic investigations, and a documented raised CSF pressure without chemical or cytologic abnormalities. These criteria are often called modified Dandy's criteria.

The condition can be divided into idiopathic (cause unknown) and secondary (subsequent to an underlying cause). In patients with an underlying cause, the condition often reverses after the predisposing factor is reversed. In benign intracranial hypertension, essentially, there is increased venous congestion in the brain, leading to brain edema associated with increased brain water content.

There have been several predisposing factors associated with this condition. Of the various associations, the following are significant: obesity; hypervitaminosis A; hypothyroidism; steroid withdrawal; medications such as Tetracycline, Danazol, oral contraceptives, and Nalidixic acid; hypoparathryoidism;

and vitamin A deficiency. It is interesting to note that both vitamin A excess and vitamin A deficiency can be predisposing factors for benign intracranial hypertension, though the association with excessive vitamin A has been more definite.

Obesity and IIH: It has been estimated that as high as 60% of men and 90% of women with BIH are obese. Weight loss, by any measure, has been shown to resolve symptoms of papilledema. Though the exact cause is unknown, it has been proposed that venous congestion may be due to reduced venous drainage from the brain due to increased intrathoracic pressure as a result of obesity. Alternatively, excessive estrogen production by the adipose tissue in obese patients may be result in IIH.

95. How do these patients present?

Of all the patients, two distinct groups can be differentiated:

a. IIH with papilledema

b. IIH without papilledema.

IIH with papilledema: This group presents with headache, nausea, transient visual obscurations, visual loss, double vision or blurred vision, and a host of nonspecific symptoms such as numbness in the extremities, ringing in the ear, shoulder and arm pain, pain behind the eyeballs, generalized weakness, and low back pain and gait instability. Headache is present in approximately 95% of patients and is behind the eyeballs and often is pulsatile. Headaches may be exacerbated by eye movements. It may be associated with nausea and less commonly with vomiting. Transient visual obscurations are usually manifested by rapid graying or blackening of the vision and may be associated with conditions that raise intracranial pressure. Blurred vision may be due to paresis of one or both the VIth cranial nerves and may be associated with inward deviation of the eyeballs. Paresis usually improves after intracranial pressure is relieved. About 25% of these patients may also have associated cognitive dysfunctions on neuropsychologic assessment. There may be associated depression, anxiety, or chronic fatigue.

On ophthalmological evaluation, there can be a host of findings due to transmission of the raised intracranial pressure to the optic nerves. This happens because the sheath surrounding the optic nerve is continuous with the intracranial compartment, thus leading the intracranial pressure to communicate with the sheath of the optic nerve. Findings include ophthalmological changes like elevation of the fundus, disc edema, and venous engorgement. Impairment of color vision and peripheral visual field loss sometimes can be early findings.

IIH without papilledema: A distinct group of patients are seen who have all these symptoms except papilledema. These constitute a relatively smaller group of patients and do not have papilledema or visual loss. The main treatment concern for these patients is managing headache.

96. How is the diagnosis confirmed?

The CT scan essentially rules out an intracranial tumor or hydrocephalus, which can present with raised intracranial pressure. Small slitlike ventricles are almost a rule than an exception.

MRI scan reveals evidence of slit ventricles with signs suggesting chronic increased intracranial pressure. MRI can also detect features of papilledema such as distension of the subarachnoid space around the optic nerve (perioptic subarachnoid space) and intraocular protrusion of the prelaminar optic nerve. The MRI scan also demonstrates empty sella in approximately 50% of patients and tonsillar descent in around 6% of patients. The MR venogram (a sequence of MRI scans that assesses the patency of the veins and is noninvasive) may be indicated to rule out a venous obstruction that can present with features similar to IIH.

Lumbar puncture: An opening pressure of more than 20 centimeters of CSF pressure is considered essential to arrive at a diagnosis. Some may consider a pressure above 25 centimeters of pressure to exclude some normal patients. Pressure is measured in lateral position, as a measurement taken in a sitting or prone position can be elevated and recorded as abnormal. The CSF examination is usually within normal limits. Abnormalities of the CSF examination essentially rule out a diagnosis of benign intracranial hypertension.

Chiari malformation and idiopathic intracranial hypertension: In Chiari malformation, there is descent of the cerebellar tonsils below the level of the rim of foramen magnum, into the upper cervical spinal canal. Now, several reports have found that patients with Chiari malformation can have papilledema (suggesting raised intracranial pressure). It has been reported that up to 5% of patients with Chiari malformation can have papilledema. However, patients with IIH can have tonsillar herniation in approximately 6% of cases. In a patient with both, it is often difficult to say whether Chiari malformation or the benign intracranial hypertension is the primary event. It is also significant when a surgery is contemplated, as lumboperitoneal shunt is relatively contraindicated with an existent tonsillar descent as seen in Chiari malformation. In such cases, the Chiari malformation is treated initially with a foramen magnum decompression, and subsequently the lumboperitoneal shunt may be considered.

97. What are the management options?

Idiopathic intracranial hypertension is often described as a *self-limiting disease* with spontaneous resolution. Spontaneous resolution can often occur within months but often it takes a year or two. The most significant concern is developing permanent visual loss that can occur in up to one-fifth of cases. Recurrence may be seen in up to 10% of cases after initial resolution. The persistence of papilledema has been reported as up to 15% of cases.

Several nonoperative and operative options have been considered in the management.

a. **Diet, weight loss, and change in lifestyle:** IA weight loss of 6% often can cause resolution of papilledema. Gastric bypass surgery as a treatment of obesity has also been considered in patients who have been unable to reduce weight.

b. **Discontinuation of offending medications:** Discontinuing offending medications should be considered in cases in which an offending medication has been identified.

c. **Acetazolamide:** Acetazolamide (Diamox) has been often the first line of management. It is reported to reduce CSF production and has been administered in doses of 500 milligrams twice or three times a day. The maximum recommended dosage is 1500 milligrams twice a day. Larger doses have reported to cause metabolic acidosis. Patients who are allergic to sulfa or have a history of renal stones cannot take acetazolamide.

d. **Furosemide:** Furosemide (Lasix), a diuretic, also has been used alone or in combination with acetazolamide.

e. **Steroids:** Corticosteroids have been used in patients with severe visual impairment as a temporary measure. Long-term steroid therapy is not recommended, as it may cause weight gain.

f. **Symptomatic treatment:** Nonsteroidal anti-inflammatory agents are often considered as the first line of symptomatic management. Antimigraine therapy often also can be started. Patients have noted improvement with amitriptyline at a lower dosage, which may be subsequently titrated for symptomatic improvement.

g. **Intermittent lumbar punctures and drainage of CSF**: Intermittent spinal taps and drainage of CSF are often beneficial in reducing the raised intracranial pressure. After a spinal tap, there can be leakage of CSF into the epidural space, which thus acts as a CSF fistula in releasing the CSF for some more days. Large bore needles (18 gauge) often have been used to facilitate this process. Serial lumbar punctures uncommonly can result in acquired tonsillar herniation. In a previous study, about one-fourth of patients had remittance of the symptoms after the initial LP.

h. **Optic nerve sheath fenestration:** Optic nerve sheath fenestration has been considered to protect from vision loss and to manage papilledema. It does not have a significant role in patients who present with headache as their predominant symptom and who do not have papilledema. In this surgery, by an approach through the orbit (eye socket), several slits are made in the sheath of the optic nerve to let out the spinal fluid. Improvement of the visual field can occur in 50–100% of patients. A repeat fenestration may be required in around 6% of cases. Sometimes bilateral fenestration may be required. As mentioned earlier, the procedure is not effective at treating symptoms like headache and raised intracranial pressure.

i. **Lumbar CSF shunting procedures:** Lumbar shunting procedures have remained as the mainstay of neurosurgical treatment of persistent headache associated with raised intracranial pressure. The temporary relief of symptoms following a lumbar puncture and its recurrence a few days later suggests possible benefit with lumbar shunting procedures. Most neurosurgeons prefer lumbar shunt to the ventricular shunt as the tiny, slitlike ventricles in these patients make it technically difficult to place ventricular catheters. Though easier to place, lumbar shunts are not without complications. The common complications include mechanical problems (breakage, disconnection, migration), overdrainage, and underdrainage. It is common to see these shunts being revised frequently for recurring headaches.

j. **Ventricular CSF shunt procedures:** Ventricular shunts have often been considered in patients who have multiple failures with lumbar shunts. As mentioned earlier, the occurrence of slitlike ventricles makes it difficult to place the shunt in the ventricular cavity. Recurrent malfunctions are more common as the small ventricles do not allow much CSF space around the ventricular catheter to prevent it from being blocked by the brain tissue. Usage of stereotactic guidance and neuronavigation is usually considered essential while placing these catheters in the ventricular cavity.

k. **Cranial decompression:** Cranial decompression in the form of subtemporal craniectomy has been considered in the past and may be considered in patients when no other option is available.

98. What about idiopathic intracranial hypertension and pregnancy?

Idiopathic intracranial hypertension is often encountered in patients who are pregnant. It can be performed under two circumstances.

Patients presenting during pregnancy: Those patients who have symptoms of IIH for the first time in their life during pregnancy, often have complete relief of symptoms in the postpartum period.

However, in patients who have an established diagnosis and become pregnant, the symptoms are often more difficult to manage. The aim is to prevent visual loss and to have symptomatic relief of headaches. Patients' high-risk pregnancies should be managed by skilled obstetricians. Serial lumbar punctures and limiting weight gain can be considered in the first trimester. Acetazolamide should not be considered in the first trimester because of teratogenecity, while it can be given in the second and third trimesters.

The effective management of idiopathic intracranial hypertension often is frustrating for the neurosurgeon. Headache and other constitutional symptoms often are somewhat difficult to treat satisfactorily and lead to multiple emergency room visits and hospital admission. A multimodality management team, including neurosurgeon, neurologist, ophthalmologist, pain specialist, and dietitian is often desirable in such cases.

PART TWENTY-ONE

Long–Term Outcome of Hydrocephalus

What is the overall outcome of hydrocephalus? How many patients lead a functional life?

What is the overall mortality from hydrocephalus? Is there an association between the cause of hydrocephalus and outcome?

99. What is the overall outcome of hydrocephalus? How many patients lead a functional life?

Overall outcome and quality of life: The outcome for children with hydrocephalus is extremely variable. A previous study reported that only 32% of children had an intelligence quotient higher than 90 and 40% had IQ lower than 70 (Hoppe-Hirsch, 1998). In another recent study in 349 children with hydrocephalus, the following were the scores in the four categories of the health surveyed: overall health 0.68, physical health 0.71, cognitive health 0.57, and social-economic health 0.72 (the score was graded from 0 to 1; 0 being the worst and 1 being the best) (Kulkarni, 2007).

This suggests that cognitive impairment appeared to be the most impaired category among the four broad categories surveyed. Although children with hydrocephalus have various types of impairments, most rate their experience above the average level, suggesting that the overall outcome of hydrocephalus has significantly improved over the past few decades. As we will see later, some categories of hydrocephalus have a poorer outcome as compared with other categories.

Gainful employment, living arrangement, and driver's license: A recent study surveying 1459 patients with hydrocephalus revealed that 57% of patients with hydrocephalus who were diagnosed and received treatment before the age of 18 months were employed, while the corresponding figure was 67% for patients diagnosed between 19 months and 12 years and 93% for the patients diagnosed after 13 years (Gupta, 2007). Between 57% and 71% of patients with hydrocephalus live independently, with the lower numbers observed in patients who were treated earlier in life (<18 months). Similarly, 60–93% of patients with hydrocephalus had driver's licenses, with the patients treated later in life having the higher percentage (93%) than the patients who were treated earlier in life (60%).

100. What is the overall mortality from hydrocephalus? Is there an association between the cause of hydrocephalus and outcome?

The mortality in patients with shunt has been reported between 14% and 38% in the literature. In a long-term follow-up study of patients treated with hydrocephalus from 1964 to 1984 with a follow-up period from 5.5 to 26 years (average 17 years), 14% of patients died during the follow-up. Of these, in 38% of the cases, shunt infections were the cause (Lumenta, 1995). However, most of the data are at least a few decades old, and with advancement in diagnostics and overall improvement in management, the realistic figures is considered to be lower.

The primary diagnosis responsible for hydrocephalus plays a dominant effect on the overall outcome in hydrocephalus. In addition, the severity of treatment-related complications also plays a significant role in the overall outcome.

Among the etiologic causes of hydrocephalus, hydrocephalus associated with Grade IV intraventricular hemorrhage, severe head injury, meningitis, myelomeningocele, Dandy-Walker malformation, and seizures all significantly lower overall performance scores, resulting in poorer outcome.

In the second category, shunt infections and number of shunt surgeries influence the overall outcome in patients with shunts. Studies have also shown that occurrence of frequent seizures, longer initial hospital stay, subsequent shunt complications, and longer driving distance from the residence to the hospital were associated with poorer outcome (Kulkarni, 2007).

Resources

Hydrocephalus Support Organizations

There are a number of support organizations at the national and international level dedicated to hydrocephalus. Some of the more prominent ones are listed below. These organizations provide support, educational resources, and networking opportunities to patients and families affected by hydrocephalus. Some hold meetings and conferences for families and publish newsletters for members.

1. Hydrocephalus Association:

Hydrocephalus Association
870 Market Street, Suite 705
San Francisco, CA 94102
Phone: 415-732-7040 / 888-598-3789
Fax: 415-732-7044
Website: www.hydroassoc.org

2. Hydrocephalus Foundation:

The Hydrocephalus Foundation, Inc. (HyFI)
910 Rear Broadway
Saugus, MA 01906
Phone: 781-942-1161
Fax: 781-231-5250
Website: www.hydrocephalus.org

3. Hydrocephalus Support Group:
Hydrocephalus Support Group, Inc.
P.O. Box 4236
Chesterfield, MO 63006-4236
Phone: 636-532-8228
Fax: 314-251-5871
E-mail: hydrodb@earthlink.net

4. National Hydrocephalus Foundation:
National Hydrocephalus Foundation
12413 Centralia Road
Lakewood, CA 90715-1653
Phone: 562-924-6666
Phone: 888-857-3434
Website: www.nhfonline.org

Related Organizations

1. Spina Bifida Association:
The Spina Bifida Association (SBA) serves adults and children who live with the challenges of spina bifida. It promotes education, advocacy, research, and service to spina bifida patients and their families.
Spina Bifida Association
4590 MacArthur Boulevard, NW, Suite 250
Washington , DC 20007
Phone: 202-944-3285 / 800-621-3141
Fax: 202-944-3295
Website: www.spinabifidaassociation.org

2. Brain Injury Association of America:
The Brain Injury Association of America (BIAA) is one of the oldest and largest nationwide brain injury advocacy organizations with a mission to be the voice of individuals living with brain injury, their families, and the professionals who serve them.
Brain Injury Association of America
1608 Spring Hill Road, Suite 110
Vienna, VA 22182
Phone: 703-761-0750
Fax: 703-761-0755
Website: www.biausa.org

Some Other Useful Websites Depicting Specific Shunt Products

1. www.hydro-kids.com:
A website maintained by Codman & Shurtleff, Inc., for children with hydrocephalus

2. www.medtronic.com/your-health/hydrocephalus:
The website for Medtronic, Inc., which makes Strata Programmable shunts

3. www.integralife.com:
Website maintained by Integra Lifesciences Corporation, makers of the Orbis Sigma flow-controlled valve

4. www.lifenph.com:
A website maintained by Codman & Shurtleff, Inc., makers of the Codman Hakim Programmable shunt dedicated to patients with normal pressure hydrocephalus

Resources

References

Blount JP, Severson M, Atkins V, et al. Sports and pediatric cerebrospinal fluid shunts: who can play? *Neurosurgery*. 2004;54:1190–1198.

Boon AJW, Tans JT, Delwel EJ, et al. Dutch normal pressure hydrocephalus study: randomized comparisons of low- and medium-pressure shunts. *J Neurosurg*. 1998;88:4980–4995.

Bradley N, Liakos AM, McAllister JP, Magram G, Kinsman S, Bradley M. Maternal shunt dependency: implications for obstetric care, neurosurgical management and pregnancy outcomes and a review of selected literature. *Neurosurgery*. 1998;43:448–460.

Chen MM, Coakley FV, Kaimal A, Laros RK. Guidelines for computed tomography and magnetic resonance imaging use during pregnancy and lactation. *Obstet Gynecol*. 2008;112:333–340.

Clarnette TD, Lam SK, Hutson JM. Ventriculoperitoneal shunts in children reveal the natural history of closure of the processus vaginalis. *Pediatr Surg*. 1998;33:413–416.

Di Rocco C, Marchese E, Velardi F. A survey of the first complication of newly implanted CSF shunt devices for treatment of nontumoral hydrocephalus: Cooperative Survey of the 1991–1992 Education Committee on the ISPN. *Childs Nerv Syst*. 1994;10:321–327.

Gupta N, Park J, Solomon C, Kranz DA, Wrensch M, Wu YW. Long-term outcome in patients with treated childhood hydrocephalus. *J Neurosurg*. 2007;106(5)(suppl):334–339.

Hoppe-Hirsch E, Laroussinie F, Brunet L, et al. Late outcome of surgical treatment of hydrocephalus. *Childs Nerv Syst*. 1998;14:97–99.

Kulkarni AV, Shams I. Quality of life in children with hydrocephalus: results from the Hospital of Sick Children, Toronto. *J Neurosurg*. 2007;107(5)(suppl):358–364.

Lee M, Wisoff JH, Abott R, Freed D, Epstein FJ. Management of hydrocephalus in children with medulloblastoma: prognostic factors for shunting. *Pediatr Neurosurg*. 1994;20:240–247.

Lockhart PB, Loven B, Brennan MT, Fox PC. The evidence base for the efficacy of antibiotic prophylaxis in dental practice. *JADA*. 2007;138(4):458–474.

Lumenta CB, Skotarczak U. Long-term follow-up in 233 patients with congenital hydrocephalus. *Childs Nerv Syst*. 1995;11:173–175.

Malm J, Kristensen B, Karlsson T, Fagerlund M, Elfverson J, Eksedt J. The predictive value of cerebrospinal fluid dynamic tests in patients with the idiopathic adult hydrocephalus syndrome. *Neurology*. 2000;55:576–578.

Marmarou A, Young HF, Aygok GA. Estimated incidence of normal pressure hydrocephalus and shunt outcome in patients residing in assisted-living and extended-care facilities. *Neurosurg Focus*. 2007 Apr 15;22(4):E1.

Milele VJ, Bailes JE, Martin NA. Participation in contact or collision sports in athletes with epilepsy, genetic risk factors, structural brain lesions, or history of craniotomy. *Neurosurg Focus*. 2006;21(4):E9.

Persson EK, Anderson S, Wiklund LM, Uvebrant P. Hydrocephalus in children born in 1999–2002: epidemiology, outcome, and ophthalmological findings. *Childs Nerv Syst*. 2007;1111–1118.

Savolainen S, Hurskainen H, Paljarvi L, Alafuzoff I, Vapalahti MP. Five-year outcome of normal pressure hydrocephalus with or without a shunt: predictive value of the clinical signs, neuropsychological evaluation and infusion test. *Acta Neurochir (Wien)*. 2002;144:515–523.

Volpe JJ. Intraventricular hemorrhage in the premature infant. Current Concepts. Part II. *Ann Neurol* 1989, 25: 109–116.

Walchenbach R, Geiger E, Thomeer RT, Vanneste J. The value of temporary external lumbar CSF drainage in predicting the outcome of shunting on normal pressure hydrocephalus. *J Neurol Neurosurg Psychiatry*. 2002;72:503–506.

Walker M, Fried A, Petronio J. Diagnosis and treatment of slit ventricle syndrome. *Neurosurg Clin N Am*. 1993;4:707–774.

Warady BA, Hellerstein S, Alon U. Advisability of initiating chronic peritoneal dialysis in the presence of a ventriculoperitoneal shunt. *Pediatr Nephrol.* 2007;4:96.

Zemack G, Romner B. Adjustable valves in normal pressure hydrocephalus: a retrospective study of 218 patients. *Neurosurgery.* 2002;51:1392–1400.

Glossary

Acquired hydrocephalus: Hydrocephalus caused by conditions that are not present at birth is known as acquired hydrocephalus. Some common conditions that cause acquired hydrocephalus are meningitis, brain tumors, head trauma, subarachnoid hemorrhage, and intraparenchymal hemorrhage.

Anterior fontanel: This is the largest fontanel, which is located just behind the forehead in the midline and is placed at the junction of the sagittal suture, coronal suture, and the metopic suture. It is diamond shaped. The fontanel allows for expansion of the brain after birth.

Antibiotic prophylaxis: This indicates antibiotics administered for prevention of infection (e.g., during surgery, during hospitalization).

Antisiphon devices: These are small devices interposed in the shunt system to prevent siphoning of the cerebrospinal fluid that often causes overdrainage.

Aqueductal stenting: A surgical procedure, usually by an endoscopic route, in which a thin tube (stent) is placed in the aqueduct across the stenosed segment to maintain the cerebrospinal fluid flow from the third to the fourth ventricle.

Aqueductal web: A form of aqueductal stenosis in which a thin web of tissue blocks the cerebrospinal fluid flow across the aqueduct.

Aqueductoplasty: A surgical procedure, usually by an endoscopic route, in which the blocked segment of the aqueduct is dilated by using a small inflatable balloon.

Arachnoid granulations: Also known as, arachnoid villi; these are small protrusions of the arachnoid (the thin second layer covering the brain) through the dura mater (the outer layer). They protrude into the venous sinuses of the brain, allowing cerebrospinal fluid to enter the bloodstream from the subarachnoid space.

Arachnoid mater: The arachnoid mater is the middle of the three membranes that cover the brain and spinal cord. It is separated from the pia mater by the subarachnoid space. It is composed of delicate, spider web–like (hence, the name) tissue and surrounds the brain and spinal cord, enclosing the cerebrospinal fluid that flows under this membrane in the subarachnoid space.

Ascites: This denotes accumulation of free fluid in the peritoneal cavity.

Basal ganglia: These are a group of nuclei situated deep in the brain that are connected with the cerebral cortex, thalamus, and other areas. Basal ganglia are related to functions such as motor control and learning.

Brain herniation: Brain herniation occurs as the brain shifts across structures within the skull usually as a result of very high intracranial pressure, which can be caused by various factors: traumatic brain injury, stroke, hydrocephalus, or brain tumor. If not treated quickly, brain herniation can be fatal.

Brain stem: This is the posterior part of the brain and is continuous with the spinal cord. This is an extremely important part of the brain as the motor and sensory connections between the brain to the rest of the body pass through the brain stem. The brain stem also contains several important nuclei that provide motor and sensory innervations to the face and neck by way of the cranial nerves. The brain stem also plays an important role in regulating cardiac and respiratory function and is responsible for maintaining consciousness. The parts of the brain stem are the midbrain, pons, and medulla oblongata.

Broca's area: Broca's area is a region of the brain in the lower and posterior part of the frontal lobe and is responsible for speech production. It is named after Paul Broca who first associated the area to speech production.

Cerebellum: The cerebellum is located in the back part of the brain below the cerebral hemispheres. The brain stem is in front of it. It is responsible for coordination and motor integration.

Cerebral aqueduct: A narrow channel that drains cerebrospinal fluid is located within the midbrain connecting the third ventricle to the fourth ventricle. Obstruction to the aqueduct, known as aqueductal stenosis, results in hydrocephalus.

Cerebral hemisphere: This is one of two halves of the supratentorial part of the brain delineated by a median fissure and the falx cerebri. The brain thus is divided into left and right cerebral hemispheres. Each hemisphere has an outer layer of gray matter (the cerebral cortex) and an inner layer of white matter. The hemispheres are joined by the corpus callosum, anterior commissure, and posterior commissure, which transfer information between the two hemispheres.

Cerebrospinal fluid (CSF): This is the clear bodily fluid present in the subarachnoid space (the space between the arachnoid mater and the pia mater) and the ventricular system. It acts as a "cushion" for the brain and provides a basic mechanical and immunologic protection to the brain inside the skull. CSF is produced in the choroid plexus.

Chiari malformation: In Chiari malformation, there is a downward displacement of the cerebellar tonsils into the upper part of the spinal canal through the foramen magnum.

Choroid plexus: Choroid plexus, a specialized cerebrospinal fluid–producing structure, is present in the lateral, third and fourth ventricles. The bulk of the choroid plexus is seen in the lateral ventricles.

Cisterna magna (large cistern): The cisterna magna is one of the largest cisterns surrounding the brain. Located between the cerebellum and the medulla oblongata (lower part of the brain stem) in the base of the brain, this communicates with the fourth ventricle by the foramen of Magendie and the foramina of Luschka.

Cisternography: A radiological study in which a contrast or a dye is placed in the cisterns by a spinal tap to study the flow of the cerebrospinal fluid.

Cisterns: These are crevices in the subarachnoid space of the brain created by a separation of the arachnoid and pia mater filled with cerebrospinal fluid. There are many cisterns in the brain.

Communicating hydrocephalus: Communicating hydrocephalus (also known as nonobstructive hydrocepha-

lus) indicates that the cerebrospinal fluid is in free communication between the ventricular system and the subarachnoid spaces. The hydrocephalus results due to impaired cerebrospinal fluid reabsoprtion in the absence of any obstruction between the ventricles and subarachnoid space. Most communicating hydrocephalus is thought to result because of functional impairment of the arachnoid granulations, which are located along the superior sagittal sinus. Some examples of the communicating hydrocephalus, include normal pressure hydrocephalus, hydrocephalus resulting from subarachnoid hemorrhage, and meningitis.

Congenital hydrocephalus: This indicates that the causes responsible for hydrocephalus were present at the time of birth or occurred sometime immediately after birth. The causes can be either genetic or acquired and usually occur within the first few months of life. Some examples of congenital hydrocephalus include intraventricular matrix hemorrhages in premature infants, infections, Chiari malformation associated with myelomeningocele aqueductal stenosis, and Dandy-Walker malformation.

Contrast-injected CT scan: This indicates that the CT scan was performed with injecting contrast (a radiographic dye that is easy to visualize in the CT scan). Contrast-enhanced CT scan is usually necessary for diagnosing tumors, infections, and blood vessel abnormalities.

Corpus callosum: Corpus callosum is a bundle of nerve fibers connecting the left and right cerebral hemispheres, thus transferring information between the two halves of the brain.

Cranial end of the shunt: This denotes the part of the shunt entering the intracranial compartment.

Craniosynostosis: Craniosynostosis is a condition in which there is premature fusion of one or more sutures in an infant skull, thus changing the growth pattern of the skull.

CSF glucose: The glucose concentration in the cerebrospinal fluid. It is considerably reduced in bacterial meningitis and helps in corroborating the diagnosis.

CSF protein: The protein concentration in the cerebrospinal fluid.

Cystoperitoneal shunt: Here the shunt is placed between the cyst (fluid cavity) in the brain and the abdominal cavity.

Dandy-Walker malformation: This is a congenital brain malformation involving the cerebellum and the fourth ventricle. The components of Dandy-Walker syndrome include absence of cerebellar vermis, obstruction of the opening of the fourth ventricle, and associated hydrocephalus. All components may or may not be present. There may be various degrees of associated developmental delay. It is considered to be a genetically sporadic disorder that occurs 1 in every 25,000 live births.

Differential pressure valves: These valves open and close according to a preset opening and closing pressure by the manufacturer. For example, when the intraventricular pressure exceeds the opening pressure, the valve opens and drains the fluid until the pressure drops below the closing pressure, thus stopping the flow.

Distal shunt obstruction: Obstruction to the cerebrospinal fluid flow occurring in the distal catheter (e.g., peritoneal catheter in a ventriculoperitoneal shunt).

Dura mater: This is the outermost of the three layers of the meninges surrounding the brain and spinal cord (the other two meningeal layers are the pia mater and the arachnoid mater). The dura surrounds the brain and extends to cover the spinal cord. The term *dura mater* is derived from Latin, indicating "tough mother," consistent with its tough and leather-like structure.

Falx cerebri: This is a strong, arched fold of dura mater descending vertically between the cerebral hemispheres. It is named for its sickle shape (narrow in front and broader behind).

Flow-regulated valve: In flow-regulated valve, the cerebrospinal fluid flows at a predetermined constant rate irrespective of the intraventricular pressure. Unlike the differential pressure valves, overdrainage due to siphoning does not occur in flow-regulated valves.

Fontanel: Fontanel are soft areas on a baby's head that are still not ossified. The two common fontanel are the anterior and posterior fontanel. The fontanel allows a quick estimation of the intracranial pressure in the early neonatal period.

Foramen of Luschka: The two foramina of Luschka are the lateral apertures, one on each side communicating the fourth ventricle to the cisterna magna. Along with the foramen of Magendie, these are the primary routes for drainage of cerebrospinal fluid out of the fourth ventricle.

Foramen of Magendie: Foramen of Magendie is the median aperture communicating the fourth ventricle to the cisterna magna.

Foramen of Monro: The foramen of Monro (interventricular foramen) is a channel that connects the lateral ventricle with the third ventricle and is located just next to the midline of the brain. It permits cerebrospinal fluid produced in the lateral ventricles to reach the third ventricle. There are two foramina of Monro, one on each side.

Fourth ventricle: The fourth ventricle is one of the four fluid-filled cavities in the brain. The fourth ventricle is located behind the brain stem in the region of the pons and medulla. Cerebrospinal fluid enters the fourth ventricle through the cerebral aqueduct and exits through two lateral foramina of Luschka and the midline foramen of Magendie to the subarachnoid space.

Frontal lobes: The frontal lobe is an area in the brain located in the front part of each cerebral hemisphere and positioned in front of the parietal lobes and above and in front of the temporal lobes.

Gram's stain: Gram's staining is a microbiological laboratory technique. The technique is used as a tool to differentiate between gram-positive and gram-negative bacteria as a first step to determine the identity of a particular bacterial sample. The word Gram refers to Hans Christian Gram, the inventor of Gram's staining.

Hydrocephalus: A medical condition in which there is an abnormal accumulation of cerebrospinal fluid in the ventricles or cavities of the brain.

Hypothalamus: The hypothalamus is the part of the brain below the thalamus that contains a number of small nuclei with a variety of functions. The hypothalamus controls body temperature, hunger, thirst, fatigue, sleep, and sleep–wake cycles.

Idiopathic intracranial hypertension (IIH): Idiopathic intracranial hypertension (IIH), also known as benign intracranial hypertension (BIH) or pseudotumor cerebri (PTC), is a condition characterized by increased intracranial pressure in the absence of a tumor or other conditions such as hydrocephalus.

Infratentorial compartment: The infratentorial compartment of the brain is the area located below the tentorium cerebelli. The infratentorial region contains the cerebellum and the brain stem.

Inion: The inion is the most prominent projection of the occipital bone at the lower back part of the skull.

Internal capsule: A region of brain composed of white matter that separates the caudate nucleus and the thalamus from the lenticular nucleus. The internal capsule contains both ascending and descending axons, which house the long tracts running between the cerebral cortex and the brain stem.

Lateral ventricle: The lateral ventricles are part of the ventricular system of the brain. There are two lateral ventricles, one on each side of the brain. They are the largest of the ventricles. The lateral ventricle connects to the central third ventricle through the foramen of Monro.

Lumboperitoneal shunt: A shunt diverting cerebrospinal fluid from the lumbar region to the abdominal cavity. Usually used as an alternative to ventriculoperitoneal shunt.

Meninges: Membranes that envelop the central nervous system. The meninges consist of three layers: the outer dura mater, the middle arachnoid mater, and the deep pia mater. The primary function of the meninges is to cover and protect the central nervous system.

Motor strip: This is a band of cerebral cortex (gray matter) running along the side of the frontal lobe of the brain that controls all bodily motor movements. It is also known as the primary motor cortex. It is located in front of the central sulcus.

Myelomeningocele: In this form of spina bifida, through a defect in the coverings of the spinal cord (either all or some of the following: meninges, muscle, bone, skin), the neural tissue (spinal cord or the nerve roots) protrude outside the confinement of the spinal canal in varying degrees, from a small defect with well-covered skin to exposed spinal cord with a flattened platelike mass of nervous tissue (myeloschisis). The exposure of the nervous tissues results in usually permanent neurologic deficits.

Nasion: The nasion lies in the intersection of the frontal the nasal bones. It is identified by the depressed area between the eyes, just superior to the root of the nose.

Normal pressure hydrocephalus (NPH): Commonly seen in elderly people, this form of communicating hydrocephalus presents with a varying combination of memory impairment, gait instability, and urinary incontinence. There is accumulation of cerebrospinal fluid not accompanied by a significant raised intracranial pressure (hence, normal pressure hydrocephalus).

Obstructive hydrocephalus: Hydrocephalus caused by an obstruction of the cerebrospinal fluid pathways. Common examples are aqueductal stenosis and tumors causing hydrocephalus.

Occipital lobe: The occipital lobe is located in the back part of the brain behind the parietal lobes and contains the visual cortex and processing center.

Parietal lobes: The parietal lobe is a part of the brain located above the temporal and occipital lobes and behind the frontal lobe. This part of the brain integrates sensory information.

Pia mater: The pia mater is the innermost layer of the three layers of membranes surrounding the brain and spinal cord. The pia mater closely envelops the entire surface of the brain running down into the fissures and the sulci of the brain.

Posterior fontanel: Fontanel are soft spots on a baby's head, which, during birth, enable the bony plates of the skull to bend, allowing the child's head to pass through the birth canal. The posterior fontanel is triangular shaped and is located at the junction of the sagittal suture and lambdoid suture. It generally closes 6 to 8 weeks after birth.

Posterior fossa tumor: Tumors located in the posterior fossa of the cranial cavity. The common tumors located in posterior fossa are medulloblastoma, ependymoma, cerebellar glioma, and intracranial metastatic tumors. These tumors commonly cause hydrocephalus by obstructing the cerebrospinal fluid pathways.

Posthemorrhagic hydrocephalus: Hydrocephalus resulting after bleeding inside the brain with the blood products obstructing the cerebrospinal fluid pathways. Common examples are hydrocephalus associated with intraventricular hemorrhage of prematurity and hydrocephalus following subarachnoid hemorrhage.

Posttraumatic ventriculomegaly: Dilatation of the ventricles following significant brain trauma. The excessive cerebrospinal fluid accumulation does not usually require a surgical intervention.

Proximal shunt obstruction: Obstruction of the shunt at the ventricular end. Common obstructive elements are the choroid plexus or brain parenchyma.

Pseudomeningocele: An abnormal collection of cerebrospinal fluid (CSF) communicating with the normal CSF surrounding the brain or spinal cord. In a pseudomeningocele, the fluid is contained in a cavity within the soft tissues and is not surrounded by a normal membrane. Most commonly following surgery of the brain or the spinal cord, or after trauma.

Pseudoperitoneal cyst: Localized fluid collection in the abdominal (peritoneal) cavity most commonly occurring because of poor absorption of the cerebrospinal fluid drained from a shunt tube.

Seizures: Also known as a "fit," seizure is defined in medical literature as a transient symptom of abnormal excessive or synchronous neuronal activity in the brain. It can vary from a wild thrashing movement with loss of consciousness (tonic-clonic seizure) or a brief loss of awareness with the surroundings. Occurrence of recurrent and unprovoked seizures is termed *epilepsy*.

Short segment aqueductal stenosis: A type of aqueductal stenosis in which the aqueduct is obstructed only for a short segment of its length.

Shunt tap: Tapping of the shunt reservoir to obtain cerebrospinal fluid for diagnostic or therapeutic purposes.

Siphoning: In neurosurgical literature, siphoning denotes excessive drainage of cerebrospinal fluid because of a difference of levels between the ventricles and the distal cavity (e.g., peritoneal cavity, pleural cavity) through the shunt tube.

Slit ventricle syndrome: A condition associated with slitlike ventricles with symptoms of overdrainage and low-pressure headache. The collapsed ventricles frequently block the proximal catheter leading to shunt obstruction. This is a developmental birth defect, resulting in unused skin, muscles, bone, and spinal cord. The extent of the open elements varies with severity. There may or may not be a fluid-filled sac surrounding the spinal cord.

***Staphylococcus epidermidis*:** It is one of the bacteria commonly found in skin as a common flora. Although it is usually nonpathogenic, it can cause infection in patients with a compromised immune system. Most infections are acquired in the hospital, as more virulent strains of the organism are commonly seen in hospitals because antibiotics and disinfectants are used. It is also a major concern for people with shunt catheters or other surgical implants, as it produces a biofilm on these devices.

Subarachnoid cisterns: These are cerebrospinal fluid–filled spaces in the subarachnoid space more commonly seen in the base of the brain. The subarachnoid spaces over the surface of the brain are prominent in elderly people as the brain shrinks.

Subdural collections: Cerebrospinal fluid or fluid collections in the subdural space (underneath the dura and above the arachnoid). Subdural collections are more prominent in elderly people as the brain shrinks.

Supratentorial compartment: The supratenorial compartment of the brain is the area located above the tentorium cerebelli. The supratentorial region contains the cerebral hemisphere.

Sutures: A suture is a fibrous joint that occurs in the skull and joins two or more bones together. The growth of the skull occurs by formation of bone at these sutures.

Temporal lobes: The temporal lobe is the region of the brain cortex located in the temporal region behind the frontal lobes, beneath the parietal lobes and in front of the occipital lobes. It is involved in hearing, comprehension of speech, long term memory and is home to the primary auditory cortex.

Tentorium cerebelli: The tentorium (tent) cerebelli (derived from cerebellum) is an extension of the dura mater separating the cerebellum from the occipital lobes. It divides the cranial cavity into two major compartments: the supratentorial (above the tentorium) and infratentorial (below the tentorium) compartment.

Thalamus: The thalamus is a midline-paired structure situated between the cerebral cortex and brain stem. It acts as a relaying station for sensation and motor signals to and from the cerebral cortex. It also participates in regulation of consciousness and alertness. The thalamus and hypothalamus surround the third ventricle.

Third ventricle: It is the part of the ventricular system located between the two thalami in the midline. It communicates with the left and right lateral ventricles by foramen of Monro and with the fourth ventricle by cerebral aqueduct.

Triventricular hydrocephalus: Commonly resulting from aqueductal obstruction, triventricular hydrocephalus results in dilatation of the two laterals and the third ventricle.

Unilateral hydrocephalus: Dilatation of one lateral ventricle results in unilateral hydrocephalus. The common cause in obstruction at one of the foramen of Monro.

Unitized distal end (shunt): Here, the valve and reservoir complex of the shunt is unitized with the distal catheter, thus reducing chances of disconnection in the follow-up period.

Valve complex (shunt): The valve complex commonly has the reservoir and the valve of the shunt system. At times, the antisiphon device is also integrated with it.

Ventricular catheter: The part of the shunt catheter that enters the ventricles. This connects to the valve complex.

Ventriculoatrial shunts: Shunts draining cerebrospinal fluid between the cerebral ventricles and the atrium (one of the chambers of the heart).

Ventriculoperitoneal shunt: Shunts draining CSF between the cerebral ventricles and the peritoneal cavity (also known as abdominal cavity). The peritoneum is the lining of the abdominal cavity.

Ventriculopleural shunt: Shunts draining CSF between the cerebral ventricles and the pleural cavity (pleura is the membrane lining the lungs).

Y connector: A connector commonly used with cerebral shunts to connect two ventricular ends (one each to the upper limbs of the Y) to a single distal end (the lower limb of the Y).

Index